PROBIOTICS

other AVI books on biochemistry and nutrition

PROBIOTICS

Edited by **GEORGE S. SPERTI**, Sc.D.

President, St. Thomas Institute
Cincinnati, Ohio

WESTPORT, CONNECTICUT

THE AVI PUBLISHING COMPANY, INC.

1971

Foreword

The teaching I received in immunity was based on the concept that immune tissue reactions were always due to antibodies, but experiments carried out in my laboratory indicated that such reactions may occur in the absence of antibodies. For example, I showed (Science 79, 172–175, 1934) that different tissues of nonimmune rabbits possessed different localizing capacities for tissue-injected foreign protein. When the protein was injected subcutaneously, the localization was three times as great as when injected intramuscularly. Also, on the injection of a foreign protein in rabbits, the localizing response of the skin to the specific protein increased from day to day during this incubation period, whereas precipitins first appeared at the end of the incubation period. Furthermore, these precipitins generally disappeared from the blood stream in about one week, while the localizing response remained for several weeks.

It is commonly assumed that, in the nonimmune animal, natural, nonspecific, fixed antibodies very likely play a role in the tissue-localizing response to injected foreign proteins. But it would seem more reasonable to assume that, in the absence of immunity, localization is basically a tissue response and not an antibody response.

In the presence of immunity, when antibodies circulate in the blood stream, tissue localization of injected specific protein, as is well-known, leads to an Arthus reaction. One might expect that Arthus reactions in different parts of the skin would be of similar intensity, presumably due to circulating antibodies. But it was observed in this laboratory (Univ. of Mich. Med. Bull. 22, 73–79, 1956) that Arthus reactions in different areas of the rabbit's skin differed markedly in intensity. The reactions to the subcutaneous injections of specific protein were very severe in the back and in the facial area, mild in the abdominal area, and practically negative in the groin. This finding also raised unanswered questions of the relation of tissue reactions to antibodies.

The concept that tissue localization to injected protein in the absence and presence of immunity may not be due to antibodies suggests that tissue cells may carry a characteristic of unicellular animals in drawing foreign particles to them. If then tissue cells may show reactions independently of antibodies, the probiotic studies discussed in this volume become understandable. Indeed, these studies, in my opinion, represent an outstanding breakthrough into a new and unexplored type of tissue defense against pathogenic organisms.

Reuben L. Kahn
Professor Emeritus of Serology,
University of Michigan,
Ann Arbor, Michigan
Department of Microbiology,
Howard University,
Washington, D.C.

Preface

St. Thomas Institute is a graduate school of scientific research. Its purpose is to foster fundamental research in the natural sciences and to determine as far as possible the basic laws governing natural phenomena.

The Institute was established as the Institutum Divi Thomae in June 1935, by His Grace, the Most Reverend John T. McNicholas, Archbishop of Cincinnati. It is governed by its own Board of Trustees and now has no official church affiliation.

St. Thomas Institute is a graduate school authorized to grant the degrees of M.S. and Ph.D. Its program is directed primarily toward the development, as outstanding research workers, of limited numbers of persons who show creative ability in science. An intensive experience in research is afforded such persons, and the formal course of studies which they receive is planned to give them a broad knowledge of the basic sciences (mathematics, physics, chemistry, and biology), as well as advanced training in their special fields.

The emphasis upon a broad training in the various basic sciences is consistent with the corresponding emphasis on cooperative research. It is felt that many of the important problems of modern science—and especially those in the borderline fields—can be solved more efficiently by coordinated attack from the viewpoints of several sciences. This we refer to as cooperative research.

The work described in this book is the result of such cooperative efforts. Although my name appears as its editor, the book is primarily a compilation of a series of published papers and theses of faculty members and students, representing a broad spectrum of sciences. Contributors to this work include:

A. J. Berger, Ph.D.
N. J. Berberich, Jr., Ph.D.
R. M. Bohrer, Ph.D.
E. S. Cook, Ph.D.
C. Coutinho, Ph.D.
M. P. Freijanes-Parada
A. Fujii, Ph.D.
L. Hamagami, M.D., Ph.D.

E. L. Hennessey, M.S.
A. D. Kenney, Ph.D.
E. F. Kohlmiller, Jr., Ph.D.
C. W. Kreke, Ph.D.
B. Kroenberg, Ph.D.
F. X. Lobo, Ph.D.
E. M. Lynch, Ph.D.
D. L. Medley, Ph.D.
A. J. Mukkada, Ph.D.
R. F. Naegele, Ph.D.
L. G. Nutini, M.D.
N. T. Perez-Vidal,Ph.D.
G. Schramm, Ph.D.
M. P. Schroeder, Ph.D.
J. Smolar, M.S.
G. S. Sperti, Sc.D.
K. Tanaka, Sc.D.
G. Thomas, M.S.
Y. Tsuchiya, Ph.D.
G. P. Walsh, Ph.D.

Appended to the Introduction are lists of the published papers and doctoral theses of the above contributors.

I am also indebted to Dr. E. V. Cowdry, Professor Emeritus of Anatomy, Washington University, and Dr. R. L. Kahn, Professor Emeritus of Serology, University of Michigan, for many helpful discussions during the preparation of this book, and I am additionally grateful to Dr. Kahn for the preparation of the Foreword.

GEORGE S. SPERTI

Contents

Introduction

This book embodies a series of researches on bodily defense against infection and disease which has been commonly referred to as natural resistance. Certain omega-amino acids and peptides have been isolated from animal tissues, identified, synthesized and proven effective prophylactically and therapeutically against a variety of organisms.

Broadly speaking, the experiments have demonstrated that bacterial resistance (which heretofore may have been referred to as "natural") can be artificially induced to a high degree. It will be seen that this resistance is totally independent of classical antibody formation resulting from the injection of a foreign protein. As far as is known, the resistance which we have observed is not based on *properdin* formation or any of the recognized immunological reactions. Its possible relation to *interferon* is not apparent; however, the subject bears further investigation.

We have found that the type of resistance to which we refer can be induced by administering the substances, either by injection or orally.

Scientists have long realized that the body has a defense against some common diseases which they have not been able to identify with antibody formation.

Dr. Stephen D. Elek (1959), in his classical treatise on *Staphylococcus pyogenes* stated:

"Too little is still known about the events occurring in infection to be able to discuss precisely the factors of natural resistance or of immunity upon reinfection . . . . The use of penicillin has shown what had been suspected for a long time—that a bactericidal effect *in vivo* determines the cure, and that the effects of toxin are of secondary importance. In natural resistance this sterilisation is brought about by the body of the patient, but the exact mode of action is still unknown."

Kahn (1956), in his work on local infections recognized the necessity of factors other than antibodies to explain localization phenomena.

It is widely recognized that a partial nonspecific immunity to some microorganisms can result from the injection of proteins not directly identifiable with the organism to which immunity has been induced. The resulting immunity, however, is not the type of resistance which is the subject of these studies since the resistance-inducing agents with which we are concerned are not proteins.

1

It is well known that certain species of animals are more resistant than others to various infectious organisms. One of the most common of these organisms is *Staphylococcus aureus*. It is also recognized that there is a wide variation in the degree of resistance to this organism among members of the same species including human beings.

Extensive researches have been conducted by Forssman (1935, 1936A, 1936B, 1938), Jaubert (1928), Rigdon (1937A, 1937B, 1939, 1940), Parker (1924), Parker *et al.* (1925), Ramon (1936, 1939), Ramon and Nélis (1934), Ramon and Richou (1937), Ramon *et al.* (1936A, 1936B, 1936C, 1936D, 1936E, 1936F, 1938), Richou (1936, 1937, 1953), and Burnet (1929, 1931), Burnet and Freeman (1932), Burnet and Lush (1935), Burnet and Fenner (1949), to mention but a few, in attempts to develop vaccines, antitoxins or toxoid preparations against this organism. Although minor successes have been reported with autogenous vaccines and toxoids, it is generally accepted that such procedure gives very little, if any, protection in the majority of cases.

In some of our early experiments (Cook and Kreke 1939A, 1939B; Cook and Walter 1941; Cook and Walsh 1944; Cook *et al.* 1938A, 1938B, 1940; Loofbourow *et al.* 1938, 1939; Nutini and Kreke 1942; Ruddy 1938; Schroeder 1945), we were able to demonstrate that substances could be isolated from cells (animal as well as yeast and bacteria) which could stimulate the metabolic processes of other cells. Certain fractions were shown to have the capacity to stimulate the growth of cells *in vitro*, while others could stimulate cellular respiration and still others glycolytic processes.

In many of our early experiments standard bacteriological media had not been supplemented with growth-essential substances to the same degree as present-day media. For this reason, it may not be correct to assume that the crude cellular fractions herein described are true growth stimulators, but may owe their activity to certain presently recognized growth essential compounds.

During the course of our experiments it was noted that when *Staphylococcus aureus* organisms were cultured *in vitro* in the presence of a substance isolated from beef spleen, which had been shown to be a metabolic stimulator of certain animal cells, the organisms changed some of their physical as well as their biochemical characteristics. These observations led us to investigate the effect of cellular extracts on the pathogenicity of the bacteria.

Some of the substances which showed a stimulatory effect on some organisms, when tested *in vitro*, showed an inhibitory effect on others under similar conditions. However, the therapeutically effective doses are usually small compared with the quantity of material needed to show inhibitory effects *in vitro*.

The cure and prevention of diseases resulting from the use of these substances, therefore, are not due to direct antimicrobial action, but rather to the action on the host or to the combined action of the substance and the host. Obviously, these substances cannot be termed antibiotic, since they do not display any direct bactericidal activity. Inasmuch as they act by increasing the defenses of the host, we have felt that a more definitive name would, of necessity, indicate their enhancement of the defense mechanism of the host. With this thought in mind we have chosen to call these substances *probiotics*.

Although this book is confined to laboratory animal experiments, a limited number of clinical tests have shown *probiotics* to be highly effective against penicillin-resistant *Staphylococcus aureus* infections in human beings.

PUBLISHED PAPERS DEALING WITH PROBIOTICS
ST. THOMAS INSTITUTE

BERGER, A.J., SCHRAMM, G., HAMAGAMI, L., and COOK, E.S. 1957. Antistaphylococcic factors in brain extract. Nature 179, 588.

COUTINHO, C., and NUTINI, L.G. 1963. Correlation between the essential amino-acid requirements of Staphylococcus aureus, their phage types and antibiotic patterns. Nature 198, 812.

KROENBERG, B., COOK, E.S., COUTINHO, C., and NUTINI, L.G. 1963A. Three antistaphylococcic factors from ox brain. Nature 198, 910.

KROENBERG, B., COOK, E.S., COUTINHO, C., and NUTINI, L.G. 1963B. Beef blood as a source for antistaphylococcal substances. J. Bacteriol. 86, 137.

MUKKADA, A.J., NUTINI, L.G., and COOK, E.S. 1969. Prophylactic effects of γ-aminobutyrylhistidine (homocarnosine) on experimental staphylococcal infections in mice. Appl. Microbiol. 18, 641.

NUTINI, L.G., and BERBERICH, N.J., JR. 1965. Effect of diet and strain difference on the virulence of Staphylococcus aureus for mice. Appl. Microbiol. 13, 614.

NUTINI, L.G., HENNESSEY, E.L., and LYNCH, E.M. 1945. Effect of various tissue extracts on the growth of colon-typhoid-dysentery organisms. Studies Inst. Divi Thomae 4, 97.

NUTINI, L.G., and KREKE, C.W. 1942. The toxic effect of splenic extracts on Streptococcus hemolyticus. J. Bacteriol. 44, 661.

NUTINI, L.G., KREKE, C.W., and SCHROEDER, M.P. 1945. Further studies on the effects of spleen extract on bacteria. J. Bacteriol. 50, 177.

NUTINI, L.G., and LYNCH, E.M. 1945. Effect of tissue extracts in controlling Staphylococcus aureus infections. Nature 156, 419.

NUTINI, L.G., and LYNCH, E.M. 1946A. Further studies on effects of tissue extracts on Staphylococcus aureus. J. Exptl. Med. 84, 247.

NUTINI, L.G., and LYNCH, E.M. 1946B. Comparative action of an extract of brain tissue and penicillin on Staphylococcus aureus infections. J. Bacteriol. 52, 681.

NUTINI, L.G., and LYNCH, E.M. 1947A. Response of penicillin-resistant strain of Staphylococcus aureus to extracts of beef brain. J. Pharmacol. 90, 313.

NUTINI, L.G., and LYNCH, E.M. 1947B. Response of penicillin-resistant strain of Staphylococcus aureus to extracts of beef brain. Federation Proc. 6, 281.

NUTINI, L.G., MUKKADA, A.J., and COOK, E.S. 1968. Susceptibility of Swiss albino mice to Staphylococcus aureus: diet and sex factors. Appl. Microbiol. 16, 815.

NUTINI, L.G., THOMAS, G., and SMOLAR, J. 1945. Effects of tissue extracts on growth of avirulent and virulent tubercle bacilli in vitro. Studies Inst. Divi Thomae, 4, 115.

SPERTI, G.S. 1963. Natural resistance to disease. Commentarii Pont. Acad. Sci. 37, 1.

TANAKA, K., TSUCHIYA, Y., BERBERICH, N.J., JR., MUKKADA, A.J., NUTINI, L.G., and COOK, E.S. 1968. Activity of homocarnosine and other compounds against staphylococcal infections in mice. Appl. Microbiol. 16, 1457.

DOCTORAL THESES DEALING WITH PROBIOTICS
ST. THOMAS INSTITUTE

NORBERT JOHN BERBERICH, JR. 1965. The Isolation, Purification, and Identification of an Antistaphylococcal Factor from Beef Tissue Extracts.

SR. RAYMOND MARIE BOHRER, S.S.J. 1965. Amino Acid Alterations in Mice as a Response to *Staphylococcus aureus* Infection and the Influence of Spleen Extract on These Alterations.

CLAUDE BERNARD COUTINHO. 1963. Cellular Components in Host Resistance. The Inter-relation between Modified Cellular Components of Animal Tissues and Natural Host Resistance.

MARIA PAZ FREIJANES-PARADA. 1960. Investigation of the Relationship between Certain Physical and Chemical Properties of Beef Brain Extract Fractions and Effects on *Micrococcus pyogenes* Var. *aureus.*

ALEXANDER DONOVAN KENNEY. 1950. Chemical Studies of Antibacterial Tissue Extracts.

ELMER F. KOHLMILLER, JR. 1960. The Effects of Beef Brain and Spleen Tissue Extracts on Experimental MM Virus.

BERND KROENBERG. 1963. Animal Tissues as a Source for Antimicrobial Factors.

FRANCIS XAVIER LOBO. 1959. A Re-evaluation of the Effects of Brain Extract on *Micrococcus pyogenes* Var. *aureus* with some Additional Fractionation Studies, Together with Special Consideration of the S 80/81 Group of Organisms.

DAVID LAWRENCE MEDLEY. 1962. Biochemical Investigation of Tissue Extracts. I. Treatment of *Staphylococcus aureus* Infections. II. Induction of Resistance to Neoplastic Development.

ANTONY J. MUKKADA. 1967. Part I. Homocarnosine and other Compounds: Antistaphylococcal Activity and Mode of Action. Part II. Aerobic Induction of Lactic Dehydrogenase in MIMA Polymorpha.

ROBERT FRANK NAEGELE. 1966. Tissue Extracts as a Source of Antibacterial, Antiviral, and Tumor Inhibiting Substances. Studies on a Respiratory Stimulating Factor in the Reduction of Drug Toxicity with Particular Reference to Kanamycin Sulfate and Nitrogen Mustard.

NELLY TERESA PEREZ VIDAL. 1960. Preparation and Chemical Studies of Tissue Extracts. I. Antistaphylococcic Extracts from Beef Spleen. II. Tumor Extracts which Induce Resistance to Tumor Development.

GUENTER SCHRAMM. 1956. Antistaphylococcic Factors in Brain Extract.

YOSHIKI TSUCHIYA. 1968. Identification and Activity of Antistaphylococcal Substances in Brain Extract.

GERALD PETER WALSH. 1962. Staphylococcal Infections—A New Approach in Therapy.

REFERENCES

BURNET, F. M. 1929. The exotoxins of Staphylococcus pyogenes aureus. J. Pathol. Bacteriol. 32, 717–734.

BURNET, F. M. 1931. The interactions of Staphylococcus toxin, anatoxin and antitoxin. J. Pathol. Bacteriol. 34, 471–492.

BURNET, F. M., and FENNER, F. 1949. The production of antibodies. Macmillan Co., Melbourne, Australia.

BURNET, F. M., and FREEMAN, M. 1932. The process of formol detoxication; experiments with purified staphylococcal toxin. J. Pathol. Bacteriol. 35, 477.

BURNET, F. M., and LUSH, D. 1935. The staphylococcal bacteriophages. J. Pathol. Bacteriol. 40, 455–469.

COOK, E. S., HART, M. J., and JOLY, R. A. 1938A. Effect of respiratory stimulating factors on endogenous respiration of yeast. Proc. Soc. Exptl. Biol. Med. 38, 169–170.

COOK, E. S., HART, M. J., and STIMSON, M. M. 1940. Proliferation promoting properties and ultraviolet absorption spectra of fractions from yeast. Biochem. J. 34, 1580–1587.

COOK, E. S., and KREKE, C. W. 1939A. Respiratory activity of a steam distillate from yeast. Studies Inst. Divi Thomae 2, 215–225.

COOK, E. S., and KREKE, C. W. 1939B. Malt combings as a source of respiratory factors for yeast and skin. Studies Inst. Divi Thomae 2, 173–178.

COOK, E. S., KREKE, C. W., and NUTINI, L. G. 1938B. Fractions from yeast which stimulate the respiration of yeast and animal tissues. Studies Inst. Divi Thomae 2, 23–37.

COOK, E. S., and WALSH, T. M. 1944. The effects of extracts of adult, embryo, and tumor tissues on the growth of yeast. Growth 8, 251–258.

COOK, E. S., and WALTER, E. M. 1941. Preparation and respiratory-stimulating activities of some fractions from beef spleen. Studies Inst. Divi Thomae 3, 39–52.

ELEK, S. D. 1959. Staphylococcus pyogenes and its relation to disease. E. & S. Livingstone, Ltd., Edinburgh, and London.

FORSSMAN, J. 1935. Studies in staphylococci. VI. The course of Staphylococcus infection in normal and immunized rabbits. Acta Pathol. Microbiol. Scand. 13, 453–458.

FORSSMAN, J. 1936A. Studies in staphylococci. VII. An active immunity against staphylococcal infections and its relation to known antibodies against staphylococci or products of these bacteria. Acta Pathol. Microbiol. Scand. 13, 459–485.

FORSSMAN, J. 1936B. Studies in staphylococci. VIII. The aspecific and specific effect of serums against staphylococci. Acta Pathol. Microbiol. Scand. 13, 486–501.

FORSSMAN, J. 1938. Studies in staphylococci. XIII. A further contribution to the understanding of the immunity to staphylococci. Acta Pathol. Microbiol. Scand. 15, 396–425.

JAUBERT, A. 1928. Staphylococcic vaccinotherapy. Importance of microbial metabolism. Presse Med. 36, 884.

KAHN, R. L., 1936. Tissue Immunity. Chas. C Thomas, Springfield, Ill.

LOOFBOUROW, J. R., CUETO, A. A., and LANE, M. M. 1939. Stimulation of tissue culture growth by intercellular wound hormones from injured tissues. Arch. Expt. Zellforsch. *22*, 607–613.

LOOFBOUROW, J. R., and MORGAN, M. N. 1938. Effect of respiratory and growth-stimulating factors from yeast and malt combings on bacterial growth. Studies Inst. Divi Thomae *2*, 113–127.

NUTINI, L. G., and KREKE, C. W. 1942. The toxic effect of splenic extracts on *Streptococcus hemolyticus.* J. Bacteriol. *44*, 661–666.

PARKER, J. T. 1924. Production of an exotoxin by certain strains of *Staphylococcus aureus.* J. Exptl. Med. *40*, 761–762.

PARKER, J. T., HOPKINS, J. G., and GUNTHER, A. 1925–26. Further studies on the production of *Staphylococcus aureus* toxin. Proc. Soc. Exptl. Biol. Med. *23*, 344–346.

RAMON, G. 1936. Production of *Staphylococcus* toxin and anatoxin. Compt. Rend. Soc. Biol. *121*, 375–379.

RAMON, G. 1939. The production of diphtheria, tetanus, and *Staphylococcus* toxin in patients with an object of obtaining the corresponding anatoxins. Rev. Immunol. (Paris) *5*, 385–404.

RAMON, G., BOCAGE, A., MERCIER, P., and RICHOU, R. 1936A. Staphylococcic anatoxin and its use in the treatment of infections due to *Staphylococcus aureus.* Presse Med. *44*, 185–188.

RAMON, G., BOCAGE, A., RICHOU, R., and MERCIER, P. 1936B. On staphylococcic immunity produced by specific anatoxin in patients with infections due to *Staphylococcus.* Experimental and theoretical studies. Practical applications. Presse Med. *44*, 281–284.

RAMON, G., BOIVIN, A., and RICHOU, R. 1938. Obtaining *Staphylococcus* toxin and anatoxin in a medium of definite chemical composition. Compt. Rend. Acad. Sci. (Paris) *207*, 466–468.

RAMON, G., BONNET, H., NÉLIS, P., and RICHOU, R. 1936C. The production of antistaphylococcus serum. Compt. Rend. Soc. Biol. *122*, 1002–1004.

RAMON, G., DJOURICHITCH, M., and RICHOU, R. 1936D. On staphylococcic immunity produced by specific anatoxin and the different antigens towards experimental staphylococcal infection. Compt. Rend. Soc. Biol. (Paris) *122*, 1160–1164.

RAMON, G., GERNEZ, C., RICHOU, R., and PANNEQUIN, C. 1936E. On the development of antitoxic immunity in the course of *Staphylococcus* anatoxin therapy in man. Compt. Rend. Soc. Biol. (Paris) *123*, 568–572.

RAMON, G., and NÉLIS, P. 1934. Experimental antistaphylococcic immunity by means of anastaphylotoxin. Compt. Rend Soc. Biol. (Paris) *116*, 1250–1252.

RAMON, G., and RICHOU, R. 1937. On experimental immunization by means of living pathogenic staphylococci. Compt. Rend. Soc. Biol. (Paris) *125*, 792–796.

RAMON, G., RICHOU, R., and DJOURICHITCH, M. 1936F. On the mechanism of the immunity produced by staphylococcic anatoxin with respect to infection by the virulent *Staphylococcus.* Experimental demonstration. Rev. Immunol. (Paris) *2*, 482–493.

RICHOU, R. 1936. Presence of *Staphylococcus* antitoxin of natural origin in the rat, horse and pigeon. Compt. Rend. Soc. Biol. *123*, 741–742.

RICHOU, R. 1937. Variations in immunity and in the production of specific antitoxin in two groups of rabbits treated with the samples of staphylococcic antitoxin. Compt. Rend. Soc. Biol. (Paris) *126*, 566–568.

RICHOU, R. 1953. Researches on antistaphylococcic immunity naturally occurring in man and in different animal species. Bull. Acad. Natl. Med. (Paris) *137*, 446–450.

RIGDON, R. H. 1937A. A study of immunity to *Staphylococcus* toxin in the albino rat. J. Lab. Clin. Med. *22*, 1141–1146.

RIGDON, R. H. 1937B. The effect of *Staphylococcus* antitoxin on rabbits given broth cultures of *Staphylococcus* intravenously. J. Lab. Clin. Med. *23*, 159–163.

RIGDON, R. H. 1939. Effect of intraperitoneal injections of *Staphylococcus* antitoxin on subcutaneous infection in mice. J. Lab. Clin. Med. *25*, 251–257.

RIGDON, R. H. 1940. *Staphylococcus* toxin: a resume. Am. J. Med. Sci. *2*, 412–431.

RUDDY, M. V. 1939. The specific action of two stimulating factors upon the respiration of yeast and liver cells. Arch. Exp. Zellforsch. *22*, 599–606.

SCHROEDER, M. P. 1945. Effect of yeast extract on the growth and respiration of *Azotobacter chroococcum*. Studies Inst. Divi Thomae *4*, 67–76.

CHAPTER 1

Preparation of Tissue Fractions (Probiotics) for Bacteriological Studies

A number of methods have been employed in the preparation of crude probiotics (tissue extracts); however, the following procedure (Staff Institutum Divi Thomae, 1947) has been found to give satisfactory and more consistent results and, unless otherwise stated, is the one generally used in all of the experiments presented herein.

Beef spleens, brains, livers, hearts, or kidneys in amounts of 5 to 6 lb, are obtained from a local abattoir on the day of slaughter. If necessary, they may be kept in the refrigerator up to 24 hr prior to use. They should not be frozen as this makes the tissue difficult to process.

EXPERIMENTAL PROCEDURES

Step 1—Cleaning and Grinding

All traces of blood, the *pia mater* or capsules, extraneous fat and larger blood vessels are removed while the organ is held under a moderately strong flow of cold tap water. The cleansed tissue is cut into pieces suitable for passing through an ordinary kitchen type meat grinder with the medium knife blade in place. Use of the fine blade makes separation of tissue and fluid, as well as precipitation of the proteins, difficult. The ground tissue is then weighed.

Step 2—Aqueous Extraction by Freezing and Thawing

An equal quantity of distilled water (1 ml per gm) is added to the ground tissue.[1] The mixture is thoroughly stirred and distributed among pans suitable for placing in the freezing chamber of a household type refrigerator. The mixture is frozen solid once (solid freezing of the mixture is essential) and thawed, a process usually requiring 24 hr.[2] The

---

[1] Drew's solution was originally used for extraction of the ground tissue. It is a modification of Locke's solution, the preparation of which is described by Drew (1922).

[2] Originally, 3 separate freezing and thawing processes were used, requiring 3 days.

9

mixture is centrifuged[3] at a moderately high rate of speed (1700 rpm) for 20 min,[4] and the solid residue discarded.

Step 3—Protein Precipitation

The protein material in the supernatant fluid (approximately 2 liters in volume) is precipitated at room temperature by adding sufficient 95% undenatured ethyl alcohol to make a concentration of 80%.[5] The 2 solutions are mixed thoroughly as the alcohol is added, 10.17 liters being required for each 2 liters of supernatant fluid.[6] The solution is allowed to stand overnight at room temperature and the cloudy mixture is then filtered through a Büchner funnel to remove the precipitated proteins.

Step 4—Concentration *in Vacuo*

The filtrate (approximately 10 liters) is concentrated *in vacuo* at 30°–55° C,[7] a process requiring 8 to 12 hr. The apparatus designed to permit an uninterrupted process is set up as shown in Fig. 1. The level of fluid in the round bottom flask is maintained at approximately 1500 ml by adjusting the vacuum and the screw clamp on the outlet tube from the reservoir. The large amount of free space above the liquid is useful when foaming occurs. When about one-third of the total volume of fluid remains to be distilled there may be considerable foaming. This is controlled by momentarily closing the tube (B) to the reservoir and admitting air to the circuit through the T-tube (C). The concentration process is continued until approximately 1500 ml of solution remains in the round bottom flask, or until greasy material begins to appear on its walls. The presence of this material makes subsequent filtration difficult.

[3] In some instances the mixture was not centrifuged, the alcohol precipitation of the protein being done in the presence of ground tissue.

[4] The 20-min period for centrifugation may be reduced to 5 to 10 min. The volume of the supernatant fluid is slightly reduced thereby.

[5] Originally, the protein precipitation was done in three successive concentrations of 50, 70 and 80% alcohol for 24 hr at each concentration, and at room temperature. For 2 liters of supernatant fluid 2105 ml of 95% undenatured ethyl alcohol is required for 50% concentration; an additional 2525 ml for 70% concentration (total volume 6.73 liters) and an additional 3442 ml for 80% concentration (total volume of mixture 10.172 liters).

[6] If the proteins are precipitated directly from the tissue and water mixture, no correction is made for the use of 95 rather than 100% alcohol, since the solid content would represent at least 5% of the volume. The volume of alcohol used in this case would be four times that of the original ground tissue and added distilled water.

[7] Originally the temperature was maintained at 45° C.

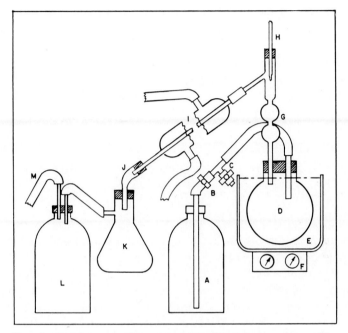

FIG. 1. DIAGRAM OF APPARATUS FOR CONCENTRATION OF EX-
TRACT IN VACUO

The reservoir (A) containing the alcoholic mixture is a 5-gal
bottle. A glass stopcock or a rubber tube with a screw clamp for
regulating the rate of flow of fluid from the reservoir connects
the outlet tube (B) through a T-tube (C) to the inlet tube in a
12-liter round bottom flask (D) supported in a water bath
(galvanized iron bucket), (E) heated by an electric hotplate
(F). The round bottom flask carries a condenser head (G), the
upper end of which is closed by a thermometer (H) in a cork
rather than a rubber stopper.[1] To the side arm of the condenser head is attached a water-jacketed condenser (I), which
is 4 ft in length, connected by an adapter (J) to a 2-liter side
arm flask (K) which, in turn, is attached by a rubber hose on
the side arm to a 5-gal waste alcohol bottle (L); through a
second tube (M) from the waste bottle, vacuum is obtained.

Step 5—Filtration to Remove Fats

Prior to its further concentration on the steam bath, the solution
removed from the round bottom flask is cooled in the refrigerator and
the congealed fatty material discarded. Passage of the solution through
a Seitz filter serves to remove more of the fatty materials. Care should

[1] A rubber stopper does not stand up as well as a cork, and it and the thermometer
may be pulled into the round bottom flask with sufficient force to break the latter.

be taken to regulate the vacuum during filtration to prevent foaming due to the fatty content of the solution.

Step 6—Concentration over the Steam Bath

Two methods for further concentration of the extract are in use, either one of which requires several days for completion. Method A: The first method consists of the evaporation of the solution in open evaporating dishes on a steam bath by continuous addition of the solution to a final volume of approximately 500 ml. The solution may be left at room temperature overnight. When the volume of 500 ml is obtained, it is divided into 100-ml lots for continued concentration to 10 ml. The sides of the dishes are scraped down carefully to prevent charring. To each milliliter of the cloudy brown viscous fluid, 2 ml of distilled water was added and the solution passed through a Seitz filter (need not be sterile) to remove the fats. Foaming should be reduced to a minimum by regulating the vacuum. The total fluid is 150 ml. Method B: The alternate procedure is to continue concentration of the solution in two large open evaporating dishes on a steam bath, the solution being added continuously during the process. As soon as the fluid in the two dishes is sufficiently reduced in volume, the two are combined in one dish and evaporation is continued to a final volume of 100 ml. Care is taken to prevent charring in the latter stages. The solid content per batch of the material prepared in this way is less than with Method A.

Step 7—pH Adjustment and Sterilization

The solutions, whether prepared by Methods A or B, are cooled, the pH adjusted to 7.0–7.1 with 10 N sodium hydroxide or concentrated hydrochloric acid using the glass electrode. The solution is then sterilized by passage through a sterile Seitz filter, precautions being taken to prevent foaming. It is then bottled in sterile rubber-capped 30-ml vials and may be stored in the refrigerator, although this latter precaution is not essential.

Step 8—Determination of Solid Content

An aliquot portion of the final solution is pipetted to a tared watch glass and evaporated to dryness in an oven at 50° to 80° C overnight. When method A is used, the solid content varies from 100 to 150 mg per ml for the total of 150 ml. When Method B is used, the range is from 125 to 175 mg per ml for the 100 ml of solution.

For bacteriological investigation in mice the extract is used without further dilution, the dose in milligrams being given on the basis of the solid content per milliliter. The check for adequate removal of protein is a negative biuret test.

REFERENCES

DREW, A. H. 1922. A comparative study of normal and malignant tissues grown in artificial culture. Brit. J. Exptl. Path. 3, 20–27.

Staff Institutum Divi Thomae. 1947. Current methods of preparation of extracts of animal tissues for use in bacteriologic and cancer investigations. Studies Inst. Divi Thomae 5, 55–64.

CHAPTER 2

In Vitro Studies of the Effects of Probiotics from Beef Spleen on *Staphylococcus aureus*

In previously published experiments (Cook and Kreke 1938A, 1938B, 1939B; Cook and Walsh 1944; Cook and Walter 1941; Cook *et al.*, 1938A, 1938B; Loofbourow and Morgan 1938; Ruddy 1938, 1939A, 1939B) we demonstrated that certain cellular extracts were capable of stimulating cellular metabolic processes including respiration, glycolysis, and growth.

The purpose of this research was to study any physical or biochemical changes which might be induced in *Staphylococcus aureus* by culturing a strain of this organism in a medium supplemented with a protein-free beef spleen extract.

The tissue extract was prepared from beef spleen using the procedure described in Chap. 1. Fifteen petri dishes divided into series of three were prepared as follows: The control consisted of a single dish containing only nutrient agar. One experimental series contained 0.5% spleen extract (pH 7.0) incorporated in the agar; the other, 1.0% of the extract. Five colonies of a two-day-old culture of S. *aureus*, isolated from the drainage of a moderately severe infection of the hand, were then inoculated into all the dishes with a fine platinum loop. At first there was apparent in all the experimental dishes a moderate depression of the colony size of the organism as compared with that of the controls. After three days of incubation, however, stimulation was noted in the dishes containing 0.5% spleen extract, and after five days, in the dishes containing 1.0% of the extract. This increase in growth over the control was manifested not only by an increase in diameter of the colonies but also by an increase in their density. The increase by surface spread was determined by tracing the individual colonies and measuring the surface area of the tracings with a planimeter. Figure 2 illustrates both the inhibitory and stimulatory effect of the extract on the organism as determined by the planimetric measurements.

Coincident with, or just prior to, the time the colony growth of the organisms in the experimental dishes was stimulated, an unexpected change in these colonies was noted. The original colonies which were implanted were uniformly orange in color and, although the control colonies continued to remain uniformly orange throughout the experiment, V-shaped wedges of white growth made their appearance in the experimental colonies at this time, gradually increasing in size, and, by the end of the sixth day, constituted almost 100% of the growth. To eliminate the possibility of any white contaminant in the original culture, organisms from the control dishes were passed through broth and plated out a number of times. This procedure resulted in the production

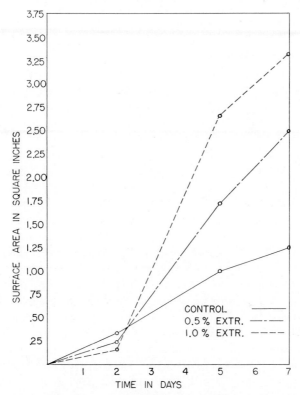

FIG. 2. EFFECT OF SPLEEN EXTRACT ON THE COLONY
GROWTH OF *Staphylococcus aureus*

of nothing other than orange colonies, thus verifying the purity of the culture. This orange organism then was inoculated into a series of petri dishes prepared as in the preceding experiment. The results were identical with those secured for the orginal orange organism, namely, initial depression of growth followed by stimulation and the appearance of white organisms in the dishes containing spleen extract.

The change from an orange to a white organism was thought at first to be an adjustment of the organism to its environment; the orange organism, being depressed in growth, reverted to the white which was stimulated. To satisfy this explanation, however, white organisms, if planted on media containing spleen extract, would necessarily have had to respond by immediate acceleration in growth, since they already had been altered to cope with the depressing effect of the extract. To test this theory, the white organism was subjected to an experiment similar in every respect to that for the orange. Instead of the expected immediate stimulation, there occurred an initial depression in growth of even greater degree and duration than that for the orange, followed by slight stimulation of about the same degree. Consequently, it cannot be assumed that the reversion of orange to white is a natural reaction to environment, but rather must be considered a change forced on the organism by the action of the spleen extract. Therefore, it must be concluded that the action of the spleen extract in the case of S. *aureus* is twofold, effecting first a change in its colony growth with initial depression and subsequent stimulation; and, secondly, a variation in its colony morphology from an orange to a white form. This variation in colony morphology, however, is not to be regarded as a distinct genetic change for, on a single passage of the white organisms through brain heart infusion broth, followed by plating on nutrient agar, a reversion to the orange was always secured. Moreover, from our own observations and those of Bigger *et al.* (1927) this variation from orange to white is a common result with old cultures and may be produced as well by the simple addition of salt (Hoffstadt and Youmans 1932) or some antiseptic dye to the medium. It is interesting to note, however, that by numerous subcultures, under the influence of spleen extract, a white organism was secured which was apparently stable and did not revert to the orange when transferred to nutrient agar.

Studies were undertaken to determine if any morphological changes had taken place in the organisms cultured in the presence of spleen extract. The results indicated that both the white and orange organisms stain uniformly Gram positive and possess normal clumping. The only difference appears to be an increase in the viscosity of the white organism cultures.

Continuing further along this line, a series of fermentation and biochemical reactions were run both on staphylococci influenced by spleen extract and on those grown normally. The results are shown in Table 1. There was no difference in the fermentation reactions except for a possible slight slowing up of the process with those organisms grown in the presence of the extract. One change in the biochemical reactions was that the organisms grown under the influence of spleen extract appeared to reduce nitrites to ammonia.

TABLE 1

COMPARISON OF FERMENTATIONS AND BIOCHEMICAL REACTIONS OF STAPHYLOCOCCI GROWN
NORMALLY AND THOSE GROWN UNDER THE INFLUENCE OF 0.5% SPLEEN EXTRACT

Fermentations	1-Day Incubation	4-Day Incubation	5-Day Incubation
Staphylococcus aureus Grown Normally			
Sugars			
Glucose...............	+	+	+
Lactose...............	+	+	+
Sucrose...............	+	+	+
Galactose.............	+	+	+
Mannose..............	+	+	+
Inulin................	−	−	−
Dulcitol..............	−	−	−
Salicin...............	−	−	−

Biochemical Reactions	5-Day Incubation
Tests	
Methyl red test...........................	+
Voges-Proskauer reaction.................	−
Nitrate reduction........................	+
Gelatin liquefaction......................	+ (?)
Indole production........................	−

Fermentations	1-Day Incubation	4-Day Incubation	5-Day Incubation
Staphylococcus aureus Grown Under Influence of 0.5% Spleen Extract			
Sugars			
Glucose...............	+	+	+
Lactose...............	+	+	+
Sucrose...............	+	+	+
Galactose.............	+	+	+
Mannose..............	+	+	+
Inulin................	−	−	−
Dulcitol..............	−	−	−
Salicin...............	−	−	−

Biochemical Reactions	5-Day Incubation
Tests	
Methyl red test...........................	+
Voges-Proskauer reaction.................	−
Nitrate reduction........................	−
Gelatin liquefaction......................	−
Indole production........................	−

REFERENCES

BIGGER, J. W., BOLAND, C. R., and O'MEARA, R. A. Q. 1927. Variant colonies of *Staphylococcus aureus*. J. Pathol. Bacteriol. *30*, 261–270.

COOK, E. S., HART, M. J., and JOLY, R. A. 1938A. Effect of respiratory stimulating factors on endogenous respiration of yeast. Proc. Soc. Exptl. Biol. Med. 38, 169–170.

COOK, E. S., and KREKE, C. W. 1938A. Fatty acids from yeast as respiratory factors. Nature *142*, 719.

Cook, E. S., and Kreke, C. W. 1938B. A note on a solid from yeast which affects cellular metabolism. Studies Inst. Divi Thomae 2, 47–49.

Cook, E. S., and Kreke, C. W. 1939B. Malt combings as a source of respiratory factors for yeast and skin. Studies Inst. Divi Thomae 2, 173–178.

Cook, E. S., Kreke, C. W., and Nutini, L. G. 1938B. Fractions from yeast which stimulate the respiration of yeast and animal tissues. Studies Inst. Divi Thomae 2, 23–37.

Cook, E. S., and Walsh, T. M. 1944. The effects of extracts of adult, embryo, and tumor tissues on the growth of yeast. Growth 8, 251–258.

Cook, E. S., and Walter, E. M. 1941. Preparation and respiratory-stimulating activities of some fractions from beef spleen. Studies Inst. Divi Thomae 3, 39–52.

Hoffstadt, R. E., and Youmans, G. P. 1932. Staphylococcus aureus. Dissociation and its relation to infections and to immunity. J. Infect. Diseases 51, 216–242.

Loofbourow, J. R., and Morgan, M. N. 1938. Effect of respiratory and growth-stimulating factors from yeast and malt combings on bacterial growth. Studies Inst. Divi Thomae 2, 113–137.

Ruddy, M. V. 1938. A note on the effect of tissue extracts upon the respiration of yeast. Studies Inst. Divi Thomae 2, 21–22.

Ruddy, M. V. 1939A. The specific action of two stimulating factors upon the respiration of yeast and liver cells. Arch. Exp. Zellforsch. 22, 599–606.

Ruddy, M. V. 1939B. A study of the respiratory activity of liver tissue in normal and vitamin-A-deficient rats. Studies Inst. Divi Thomae 2, 165–172.

CHAPTER 3

In vitro and in vivo Studies of Probiotics on Staphylococcus aureus

Extensive research has stressed the toxigenic potentiality of various strains of *Staphylococcus aureus,* demonstrating among the manifold effects of this organism its capability of producing dermonecrosis, hemolysis, and death.

The general opinion, among those who have surveyed the peculiar trends of bacteria, is that chromogenesis and other characteristic activities of these one-celled organisms will evidence themselves only when the environment is most favorable. As stated previously, this has been demonstrated with S. *aureus* in the conversion of the virulent normal S yellow colony to the avirulent white R configuration by providing unfavorable conditions for growth with the simple addition of certain dyes and salts to the media. This modification was temporary and passage *in vivo* inevitably resulted in the reversion of the variant form to the original type of colonial growth.

In preliminary experiments conversion *in vivo* was produced by injection of brain extract into animals inoculated with the yellow S organism. These findings led us to conduct the present more extensive investigations of brain and spleen extracts, as well as of heart and kidney extracts. The studies include (a) determination of the pathogenicity of the variant of S. *aureus;* (b) the prevention and treatment of staphylococcic infections with the various extracts, using different methods of inducing infection and of administering the extracts; (c) a study of the mechanism of the action of the extracts both on toxin production by the organism and on the toxin; and (d) determination of the acute and chronic toxicities of the extracts.

EXPERIMENTAL

Comparison of Pathogenicity of S and R Forms of Staphylococcus aureus

In Vitro Studies.—Aqueous extraction followed by alcohol precipitation of heart and kidney tissues from beef was made according to our original procedure described in Chap. 1 for spleen and brain, except that distilled water was substituted for Drew's solution. Extracts of the four organs, prior to further use, were checked for conversion activity *in vitro* on a virulent strain of *S. aureus* cultured from an infected tonsil. The results with all of the extracts were typical of those described in previous experiments.

In a series of three experiments, the various tissue extracts were added in concentrations of 0.5 and 1% to the solid nutrient media. Compared with the control plates, as previously observed, there was initially a slower growth rate of the inoculant, and a decrease in the size of the colonies. In the experimental plates this was followed at the end of 3 days by markedly increased growth (emanating from the original area of inoculation) of a white variant which within 2 days was approximately 3.5 to 6 times greater in area than in the control plates. The effects were most marked with brain extract.

A series of tests, designed to distinguish between pathogenic and non-pathogenic strains of *S. aureus*, were conducted in triplicate on both the S and R forms. From the data in Table 2 it would appear that the white R variant is nonpathogenic. Tests for chromogenesis made at intervals during 2½ yr show that the variant has never reverted to the original orange growth. Although none of the applied *in vitro* tests serves as a standard whereby a line of demarcation between virulence and avirulence can be drawn, some investigators maintain that negative reaction to a combination of these tests is a fairly accurate indication of non-pathogenicity (Blair 1939; Chapman *et al.*, 1934, 1937A, 1937B, 1938; Cowan 1938; Cruickshank 1937; Dudgeon *et al.*, 1928; Holman 1935; and Pinner and Voldrich 1932).

In Vivo Studies.—To determine whether the avirulence of the white R variant could be maintained *in vivo*, mice (3 to 6 months of age) BBC strain, and albino, were used as test animals. From the 3- to 5-day old experimental plates, yellow organisms were obtained from the center of the inoculation area and white organisms from the stimulated outgrowth of this area. Each test animal was injected immediately, sub-

TABLE 2

TESTS FOR DISTINGUISHING BETWEEN VIRULENT AND AVIRULENT FORMS OF *S. aureus*

Test	Control—Yellow Organism	Experimental Grey-White Organism
Fermentation of mannitol	+	−
Liquefaction of gelatin	+	+ very slight
Chromogenesis	+ yellow	− grey white
Hemolysis	+	−
Coagulase	+	−

cutaneously, with 1 ml of saline containing 1 loopful of the organisms. The experiments were made in triplicate using 10 animals for the yellow and 10 for the white organisms in each experiment. Three days after being injected with the yellow organism the control animals developed a gradually ascending paralysis, with 70% mortality by the fourth day. The remaining 30% developed large abdominal abscesses and sloughs which persisted for 3 weeks. There was no mortality among the experimental animals receiving the white organisms. These animals did not develop paralysis, and only 20% had small nonsuppurative hemorrhagic abdominal lesions which disappeared by the seventh day.

Cultures from the lesions in the survivors in each of the two groups of animals revealed organisms corresponding in type to those injected, evidence for the maintenance of the relative avirulence *in vivo* of the white *R* variant of the strain of *S. aureus* used in these experiments.

Treatment of Staphylococcic Infections with Tissue Extracts

Procedure: Control Animals.—In the following experiments extending over a period of 18 months, BBC and albino mice of the Rockland strain, 3 to 6 months of age, were used. The strain of *S. aureus* employed was obtained from the drainage of an infection on the hand and the organisms were maintained in nutrient broth as culture medium. At the time of use for injecting mice, saline suspensions were prepared with one loopful of a 48-hour culture of the organism per cubic centimeter of saline. The LD_{50} was 0.35 cc. Lesions developed within one to three days following subcutaneous injection into the ventral adbominal region and the surviving animals required 9 to 30 days to heal. Abscess formation was followed by extensive sloughing and the appearance of signs of toxification, listlessness, inability to eat, shaggy hair, cyanosis, paralysis of the limbs, and death within 5 to 6 days. Blood cultures made from animals dying showed that death was due to the *Staphylococcus*.

Following intraperitoneal (0.25 and 0.5 cc) or intravenous (0.1 cc) injection of the organisms, there were no localized lesions; a general reaction occurred characterized by roughened fur, listlessness, sluggishness, and reduced activity. Death occurred in these animals within 24 hr, and in some instances within a few minutes, following the injection. The survivors required 14 or 15 days for recovery.

Experimental Animals, Brain-extract-treated.—Brain extract was given subcutaneously in the ventral abdominal region each day to mice for: (1) prophylactic experiments, 2 to 6 hr prior to infection with *S. aureus;* and (2) therapeutic experiments, on the first day lesions developed following subcutaneous inoculation. This usually occurred after 1 to 3 days. In the case of intravenous and intraperitoneal infection, injection of the extract was given following the onset of the generalized reaction. Treatment was given daily in 50-mg doses until the lesions healed completely as judged by scabs dropping off, leaving smooth new skin beneath, or until the animals appeared normal following a generalized reaction.

In the therapeutic experiments, the animals were divided into control and experimental groups only after the lesions or the generalized reaction occurred in order to have animals with infections of similar degree of severity in each group.

The oral effectiveness of brain extract was tested both therapeutically and prophylactically using 300 mg per 24 hr, administered at intervals of 6 hr, through a curved blunt-tip hypodermic needle.

In another series of experiments the relative effectiveness of decreasing amounts of the brain extract was tested against staphylococcic infections with dosages of extract ranging from 50 mg to 5 mg daily in both a prophylactic and therapeutic series.

The control animals were injected each day with a volume of saline equivalent to that of the brain extract.

Results

In 25 experiments (Table 3), using 50 mg of brain extract daily in the prophylactic treatment of subcutaneous staphylococcic infections (227

TABLE 3

EFFECT OF BRAIN EXTRACT ADMINISTERED SUBCUTANEOUSLY AS PROPHYLAXIS AGAINST SUBCUTANEOUS *Staphylococcus aureus* INFECTIONS IN MICE

Experiment No.	No. Mice	Mortality	Lesions—Survivors		
			Average Day Appeared	Frequency	Healing Time Average (Range)
		%		%	Days
5314 BP	10C	60	3	100	12 (2 unhealed 14th day)
	10E	0	8	60	4 (3–6)
6194 BP	9C	44	6	100	17–25
	9E	0	9	55	7 (6–8)
7134 BP	10C	70	5	100	10
	10E	0	5	20	3
3265 BP	10C	100	—	—	—
	10E	0	4	50	9 (4–11)
545 BP	10C	80	3	100	22
	10E	0	2	20	6 (5–7)
1105 BP	6C	33	2	100	16 (15–20)
	6E	0	2	33	8 (7–9)
355 BP	6C	33	3	100	28 (27–30)
	6E	0	4	50	8 (5–11)
3125 BP	6C	100	—	—	—
	6E	0	3	100	7 (6–11)

TABLE 3—*Continued*

Experiment No.	No. Mice	Mortality	Lesions—Survivors		
			Average Day Appeared	Frequency	Healing Time Average (Range)
		%		%	Days
545 BP	10C	70	3	100	21 (18–23)
	6E	0	3	100	8 (5–10)
6255 BP	6C	83	2	100	20
	6E	0	2	67	9 (7–13)
625 BP	6C	83	2	100	23
	6E	0	2	67	5 (3–6)
1105 BP	6C	33	2	100	18
	6E	0	2	67	7 (5–9)
2195 BP	10C	60	3	100	17 (10–25)
	10E	0	4	50	6 (4–9)
5255 BP	10C	70	3	100	17 (12–21)
	10E	0	3	60	8 (4–10)
1025 BP	10C	100	—	—	—
	10E	0	2	50	8 (6–10)
9115 BP	10C	70	2	100	15 (9–20)
	10E	0	2	60	5 (3–8)
10115 BP	10C	90	2	100	22
	10E	0	2	50	5 (4–8)
10245 BP	6C	100	—	—	—
	6E*	0	2	83	5 (4–6)
11145 BP	10C	100	—	—	—
	10E	0	2	80	6 (4–8)
11145 BP	10C	90	2	100	25
	10E	0	3	50	6 (3–10)
11305 BP	10C	90	3	100	Unhealed on 20th day
	10E	0	3	90	7(3–11)
12105 BP	10C	80	2	100	20 (1 unhealed on 21st day)
	10E	0	2	60	7 (4–10)
12105 BP	6C	67	2	100	9 (1 unhealed on 11th day)
	6E	0	2	60	8 (6–10)
5255 BP	10C	40	3	100	19 (16–22)
	10E	0	3	70	12 (8–14)
6255 BP	20C	95	3	100	17
	20E	20	7	100	6 (3–8)
Totals and....	227C	75.0	3	100	18 (9–30)
averages....	223E	0.9	3	63	7 (3–14)

Prophylactic dose of 50 mg brain extract subcutaneously given 2 to 6 hr prior to inoculating with virulent *Staphylococcus aureus*, 1.5 LD₅₀ subcutaneously. Treatment continued at 50 mg level daily until lesions completely healed, as gauged by the loosening of the scab beneath which was a shining new intact skin surface.

* Animals ill. No open lesions; local inflammatory reaction; regression in 5 days.

control and 223 experimental mice), 25% of the controls survived the infection, and all developed typical abscesses which required from 9 to 30 days to heal. The incidence of lesions in the 99% surviving experimental animals was 63%. The interval between injection of the organisms and the appearance of the abscesses was not significantly altered in the experimental animals. The abscesses, however, were atypical in appearance, consisting of small dry lesions which did not progress to the sloughing stage and which healed completely in time intervals ranging from 3 to 14 days. There was no paralysis nor manifestations of toxic symptoms in the treated animals.

In 11 therapeutic experiments using a total of 116 control and 116 experimental animals (Table 4), treatment was begun with 50 mg of brain extract daily after the development of typical lesions following subcutaneous injection of *S. aureus*. Eighty-seven percent of the control animals and 3% of the experimental animals died. The range of healing time for the surviving control animals was 14 to 26 days with typical toxic manifestations; for the experimental animals 4 to 15 days with the absence of symptoms of toxicity.

The results of treating intraperitoneal infections in 50 mice by subcutaneous injection of 50 mg of brain extract per day, both prophylactically and therapeutically, are shown in Table 5. In the prophylactic

TABLE 4

THERAPEUTIC RESPONSE OF MICE WITH SUBCUTANEOUS *Staphylococcus aureus* INFECTION TO SUBCUTANEOUS TREATMENT WITH BRAIN EXTRACT

Experiment No.	No. Mice	Mortality	Survivors Healing Time Average (Range)
		%	Days
10194 BT	10C	100[1]	—
	10E	0	8 (7–13)
625 BT	10C	100	—
	10E	0	8 (6–9)
1295 BT	6C	83	23
	6E	0	9 (7–12)
755 BT	10C	50	16 (1020)[2]
	10E	0	6 (4–9)
9115 BT	10C	80	18 (14–22)
	10E	0	8 (4–12)
9295 BT	10C	100	—
	10E	0	7 (5–10)
10115 BT	10C	100	—
	10E	0	8 (4–11)
11145 BT	10C	100	—
	10E	10	7 (4–9)
11165 BT	10C	70	18 (15–21)
	10E	0	9 (6–13)
525 BT	10C	80	25 (23–26)
	10E	0	10 (4–15)
6255 BT	20C	95	14
	20E	15	9(6–13)
Totals and.......	116C	87	19 (14–26)
averages.......	116E	3	8 (4–15)

Subcutaneous dose of *Staphylococcus aureus* equivalent to approximately 1.5 LD$_{50}$.

Treatment begun only when all animals had open lesions, usually on 2nd or 3rd day after injection with 1.5 LD$_{50}$ of *Staphylococcus aureus* and continued until complete healing occurred, using 50 mg of brain extract subcutaneously once daily.

[1] Mortality 80% at 21 days, 100% at end of 6 weeks, due to secondary outbreaks of infection.

[2] One unhealed on 22nd day.

TABLE 5

RESPONSE OF MICE TO SUBCUTANEOUS INJECTIONS OF BRAIN EXTRACT AS PROPHYLACTIC
AND THERAPEUTIC TREATMENT OF INTRAPERITONEAL INFECTIONS WITH *Staphylococcus
aureus*

| Experiment No. | No. Mice | Mortality | Survivors—Illness | | |
			Day of Onset	Frequency	Recovery Time Average (Range)
			Prophylaxis		
		%		%	Days
1185 BP	10C	100	—	—	—
	10E	10		No illness manifested	
2185 BP	10C	40	3	100	14 (14)
	10E	0	3	100	3 (3)
11244 BP[1]	10C	80	1	100	23 (23)
	10E	0	1	100	8[4] (8)
Totals and..	30C	67	2	100	19 (19)
averages..	30E	3	2	100	6 (6)
			Therapeusis		
11154 BT[2]	10C	100	—	—	—
	10E	0	1	100	3 (3)
11154 BT[3]	10C	100	—	—	—
	10E	0	1	100	5 (5)
Totals and..	20C	100	—	—	—
averages..	20E	0	1	100	4 (4)

[1] All surviving control animals developed abscesses at site of injection; 3 experimental animals had slight sloughs at site of injection which healed within 11 days.

[2] 0.25 cc inoculant used. Experimental animals treated for 10 days.

[3] 0.5 cc inoculant used.

[4] Dry slough appeared at site of injection on day 9 in 3 animals; healed 11 days later.

series, 20 of the 30 control animals died and the survivors required 14 to 23 days to recover from the generalized reaction. Of the 30 experimental animals receiving a single preliminary dose of 50 mg of brain extract subcutaneously, followed by 50 mg per day, one died (1185 BP; the other 9 animals in this group did not react to the injection of the organisms in any apparent way) and the 20 remaining experimental animals seemed normal again within 3 to 8 days. In the therapeutic series, none of the 20 control animals survived the intraperitoneal injection of organisms while 100% of the experimental animals survived and appeared to be completely recovered within 3 to 5 days.

Of the 35 experimental animals receiving *S. aureus* injections intravenously (Table 6) and treated with brain extract subcutaneously, whether prophylactically or therapeutically, none died. The single survivor of the 35 control animals required 15 days for recovery from the generalized reaction. Three, 4 and 6 days were required for recovery of the experimental animals with the exception of 1 group which had

TABLE 6

RESPONSE OF MICE TO SUBCUTANEOUS INJECTIONS OF BRAIN EXTRACT AS PROPHYLACTIC
AND THERAPEUTIC TREATMENT OF INTRAVENOUS INFECTION WITH *Staphylococcus
aureus*

Experiment No.	No. Mice	Mortality	Survivors—Illness		
			Day of Onset	Frequency	Recovery Time Average (Range)
			Prophylaxis		
		%			Days
195 BP	10C	100	—	—	—
	10E	0	1	100	3 (2–3)
10205 BP	9C[1]	100	—	—	—
	9E[2]	0	Immediate reaction of all animals with improvement in 15–30 min.		
			Therapeusis		
195 BT	10C	100	—	—	—
	10E	0	Immediate	100	6 (4–8)
213 BT	6C	83	1	100	15 (15)
	6E	0	1	100	4 (3–4)

Animals inoculated with 0.1 cc of a 24 hr culture of organism.
[1] All dead within 24 hr of inoculations.
[2] Treatment continued for 3 days.

been treated prophylactically (10205 BP). In this group there was an immediate generalized reaction of all of the animals to the intravenous injection, but within 15 to 30 min all had apparently recovered. Treatment was continued for three days in this group. All of the control animals died within 24 hr after inoculation.

In Table 7 are given the results of using doses of brain extract graded to as low as 5 mg per day prophylactically in a series of 6 groups of 6 experimental animals each, and 1 group of 6 control animals. There was no mortality among the experimental animals until the amount of brain extract was reduced to 10 and 5 mg per day, while the healing time was gradually lengthened with the daily administration of smaller amounts. The single surviving control animal required 23 days for the healing of the lesion.

In the therapeutic experiments of the same series, there were no deaths in the 6 groups of 10 experimental animals each, while all of the 10 control animals died. The healing time with this, as with the prophylactic series, was lengthened gradually as the daily amount of brain extract injected was reduced.

The oral effectiveness of brain extract therapy for subcutaneous S. *aureus* infections is demonstrated by the data in Table 8. None of the treated animals in either the prophylactic or the therapeutic series died, while all of the controls for the therapeutic series died. There were two

TABLE 7

EFFECT OF VARIOUS SUBCUTANEOUS DOSES OF BRAIN EXTRACT ON SUBCUTANEOUS
Staphylococcus aureus INFECTIONS IN MICE

Dosage, *mg/day*	50[1]	40	30	20	10	5	Controls
	Prophylactic						
No. mice	6	6	6	6	6	6	6
Mortality, %	0	0	0	0	16	33	83
Survivors							
Average day for lesions	2	2	2	2	2	2	2
Frequency, survivors, *per cent*	67	67	83	100	100	100	100
Healing time, average, *days*	5	5	8	6	9	10	23
Range, *days*	(3–6)	(4–8)	(4–11)	(4–10)	(5–15)	(8–13)	—
	Therapeutic[2]						
No. mice	10	10	10	10	10	10	10
Mortality, %	0	0	0	0	0	0	100
Survivors							
Healing time, average, *days*	7	7	11	9	11	11	—
Range, *days*	(5–10)	(4–10)	(3–17)	(5–13)	(8–13)	(7–13)	

[1] Data included in both Tables 3 and 4.

[2] Abscesses in 100% control and experimental animals on 4th day following subcutaneous inoculation of *Staphylococcus aureus*. Brain extract therapy was begun daily on day 4 and continued until complete healing occurred as defined in Table 3. Dose of inoculant 1.5 LD50.

surviving controls in the prophylactic series requiring 15 to 21 days for healing of the abscesses. In the ten experimental animals receiving a single prophylactic dose of 300 mg of brain extract *per os* only one developed an abscess, which appeared five days after subcutaneous infection with *S. aureus*. Lesions developed in all of the control animals of this series on the second day after infection.

TABLE 8

RESPONSE OF MICE WITH SUBCUTANEOUS *Staphylococcus aureus* INFECTIONS TO 300 MG
PER DAY OF BRAIN EXTRACT ADMINISTERED ORALLY

Experiment No.	No. Mice	Mortality	Lesions—survivors		
			Average Day Appeared	Frequency	Healing Time Average (Range)
		Prophylaxis			
		%		%	Days
2195 BP	10C	80	2	100	18 (15–21)
	10E	0	5	10	5 (5)
		Therapeusis			
3265 BT	10C	100	—	—	— —
	10E	0	1	100	8 (4–11)
Totals and	20C	90	2	100	18 (15–21)
averages	20E	0	3	55	7 (4–11)

Brain extract administered at intervals of 4 hr through a curved needle directly into the stomach, a total of 300 mg per day being given. *Staphylococcus aureus* dose was 1.5 LD50.

Other Tissue Extracts.—Prophylactic and therapeutic tests on sub-cutaneous infections with the other beef tissue extracts—liver, spleen, heart, and kidney—were accompanied by results less striking than those with brain extract. In the prophylactic tests only the spleen-extract-treated animals showed significant results. These compared favorably with those for brain extract in that there was no mortality among the animals and only a slightly more prolonged healing time for lesions (Table 9). In the therapeutic experiments there was no mortality when the spleen and heart extracts were used, but a slightly longer time (7 to

TABLE 9

RESPONSE OF MICE TO PROPHYLACTIC AND THERAPEUTIC SUBCUTANEOUS ADMINISTRATION OF LIVER, HEART, KIDNEY, AND SPLEEN EXTRACTS FOR CONTROL OF *Staphylococcus aureus* INFECTIONS IN MICE

	Liver		Heart		Kidney		Spleen	
	Control	Experimental	Control	Experimental	Control	Experimental	Control	Experimental
Prophylaxis								
No. mice	6	6	10	10	10	10	6	6
Mortality, %	67	83	50	60	60	10	33	0
Survivors-lesions								
Average day of appearance	2	2	1	2	1	2	2	2
Frequency, %	100	100	100	100	100	55	100	67
Healing time, average	16	22	15	13	15	9	18	8
Range	(16)	(22)	(14–15)	(12–16)	(14–17)	(8–9)	(18)	(7–8)
No. mice			6	6	6	6	6	6
Mortality			33	0	33	17	83	0
Survivors-lesions								
Average day of appearance			2	2	2	2	2	2
Frequency, %			100	83	100	83	100	100
Healing time, average			18	8	18	11	23	10
Range			(18)	(5–13)	(18)	(7–15)	(23)	(10)
Totals and averages for prophylactic experiments — No. mice	6	6	16	16	16	16	12	12
Mortality	33	83	45	40	50	13	44	0
Healing time	4	—	18	10	17	10	21	9
Range	(4)		(18)	(5–11)	(14–18)	(8–15)	(18–23)	(7–10)
Therapeusis								
No. mice	6	6	6	6	6	6	6	6
Mortality	83	83	83	0	83	83	83	0
Survivors-lesions								
Average day of appearance	2	2	3	3	1	1	1	1
Frequency, %	100	100	100	100	100	100	100	100
Healing time, average	23	25	23	10	23	11	23	11
Range	(23)	(25)	(23)	(7–14)	(23)	(11)	(23)	(8–12)

Subcutaneous infections induced with 1.5 LD₅₀ *Staphylococcus aureus*.

14, and 8 to 12 days, respectively) was required for complete healing of the lesions than was the case with brain extract (3 to 15 days). (Table 9, Fig. 3). The infection in animals treated with kidney extract, however, showed but slight improvement as compared with that of the controls. It was felt that the poor results in this case may have been due in some measure to the toxicity of the extract at the dosage used, since all animals treated with the kidney extract exhibited toxic manifestations immediately following injection of the material. The liver extract proved too toxic to warrant further investigation.

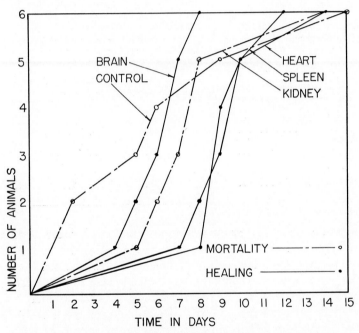

FIG. 3. COMPARISON OF THERAPEUTIC ACTION OF BRAIN, SPLEEN, HEART, AND KIDNEY EXTRACTS ON STAPHYLOCOCCIC INFECTIONS INITIATED SUBCUTANEOUSLY

Extracts and Toxin Production.—Control tubes containing nutrient broth, and experimental tubes containing nutrient broth plus 1% brain extract, were inoculated with *S. aureus* and allowed to incubate for 48 hr. Both sets of tubes were then centrifuged slowly for 15 min at the end of which time the supernatant materials were subjected to several filtrations through Berkefeld filters.

To determine whether brain extract prevented the formation of toxin by *S. aureus*, the experimental and control filtrates were injected into test mice. The control filtrate was divided into 2 parts, and 1% brain extract was added to 1 portion to eliminate any variable which might have been introduced by the presence of brain extract in the experimental filtrate. In 2 series of experiments 3 groups of 10 mice each were injected subcutaneously in the abdominal region with 0.5 ml of each of the filtrates. Observations on necrosis, hemolysis, and death are recorded in Table 10. The control filtrate was markedly toxic both as to its power to necrose tissue and to produce hemolysis, while that prepared from organisms grown under the influence of brain extract was practically nontoxic. It is apparent from the data presented that the hemolytic

TABLE 10

EFFECT OF BEEF BRAIN EXTRACT ON THE TOXIN PRODUCTION BY *Staphylococcus aureus* AS TESTED IN MICE

Type of Filtrate	Mortality	Average Hemo-globin 4th Day of Infection	Average RBC 4th Day of Infection	Necrosis
	%	%		
Toxin filtrate of *Staphylococcus aureus*, control.............	100	23.4	2,136,000	10, severe
Toxin filtrate of *Staphylococcus aureus*, control plus extract..	60	54.0	4,448,000	5, moderate 5, slight
Toxin filtrate of *Staphylococcus aureus*, experimental.......	10	91.2	9,625,000	2, slight 8, none

Ten mice in each series, weight of animals 20 gm.

and necrotic effects of toxin, while not eliminated, were considerably reduced by the simple addition of brain extract to the control filtrate.

To check for the lethal action of the toxin of S. *aureus*, 3 groups of 10 mice each were inoculated intravenously with the 3 filtrates, each mouse receiving 0.5 ml. There was almost immediate total mortality of the animals receiving the control filtrate and those receiving the control filtrate to which brain extract had been added, but there were no ill effects in those animals injected with the filtrate from organisms grown in the presence of brain extract.

The cholesterol content of the extract was 0.032 mg per dose and the phospholipid content was too small to determine. The content of these substances is too small to account for the action of the extract against the strain of S. *aureus* used. Preliminary experiments indicate that the protection by the extracts against the infection is not due to a nonspecific effect such as leukocytosis. Apparently, therefore, the effectiveness of brain extract in combatting S. *aureus* infections in animals may be due, at least in part, to its action in preventing toxin formation and to its action on the formed toxin itself.

Toxicity of Extracts.—Since previous experiments indicated that extracts of brain and spleen were less toxic than those of heart and kidney, slightly higher dosage levels of the former were used in acute toxicity tests. The results demonstrate the greater toxicity of the heart and kidney extract (Table 11). Doses smaller than 500 mg of brain and spleen extract, a dosage approximately equivalent to 2 to 2.5% of the body weight, did not kill the animals. Injections of the spleen extract were accompanied by evidence of toxicity in the form of weight loss. Heart and kidney extracts, in addition to producing marked weight loss, resulted in mortality with dosages as low as the 80 mg level, an amount equal approximately to 0.3% of the body weight.

The tests for chronic toxicity (Table 12) likewise showed brain and spleen extracts to be safer materials. The low mortality in animals receiving brain extract occurred only within the last few days of the 60-day experiment. Mortality from the use of spleen and heart extracts was greater than with brain, and occurred in the third quarter of the experimental interval. Mortality with the spleen extract was somewhat lower than that for the heart extract even though it was given at a higher dosage level. The kidney extract produced 100% mortality with both dosages within 40 days after beginning injections.

SUMMARY

(1) The ability of alcoholic-precipitated extracts of beef tissue—brain, spleen, heart, and kidney—to stimulate the growth of S. *aureus, in vitro,* and to convert the yellow S form to a white R variant with altered biochemical characteristics conforming to those of an avirulent organism, has been established.

(2) The avirulence of the white R variant has been established by *in vivo* tests on mice.

(3) Mice inoculated with *Staphylococcus aureus* subcutaneously, intraperitoneally, and intravenously, responded favorably when treated with brain extract prophylactically or therapeutically, either subcutaneously or orally.

(4) The extracts appeared equally efficient when used therapeutically (mortality 2% of 162 experimental animals and 90% in the control series), or prophylactically, (mortality 2% of 282 experimental animals and 76% in 286 control animals). The mortality of the combined prophylactic and therapeutic groups was 2% in 444 experimental animals and 81% in 448 control animals.

(5) Extracts of brain and spleen were more effective than those of either heart or kidney.

TABLE 11
ACUTE TOXICITY OF BEEF TISSUE EXTRACTS IN MICE OVER A 10 DAY PERIOD

Type of Extract	No. Mice[1]	Mortality at Different Dosages[2]						Average Weight Gain or Loss					
		50 Mg	100 Mg	200 Mg	300 Mg	400 Mg	500 Mg	50 Mg	100 Mg	200 Mg	300 Mg	400 Mg	500 Mg
		%	%	%	%	%	%	Gm	Gm	Gm	Gm	Gm	Gm
Brain.........	12	0	0	0	0	0	100	+1.3	+1.15	+1.6	+0.8	+1.25	—
Spleen........	12	0	0	0	0	0	100	−0.8	−0.2	+0.9	−1.1	−1.6	—

Type of Extract	No. Mice[1]	20 Mg	40 Mg	80 Mg	140 Mg	200 Mg	20 Mg	40 Mg	80 Mg	140 Mg	200 Mg
Heart.........	10	0	0	50	50	50	−0.1	+0.15	−1.2	−1.0	−3.2
Kidney........	10	0	0	50	50	0	−0.9	−1.7	−1.9	−0.9	−6.3

[1] Average weight, 20 gm.
[2] Daily injections, subcutaneously.

TABLE 12

CHRONIC TOXICITY OF BEEF TISSUE EXTRACTS IN MICE OVER A 60-DAY PERIOD

Type of Extract	No. Mice[1]	Extract Dosage[2]	Average Weight Gain	Experimental Interval Before Death	Mortality
		Mg	Gm	Day	
Brain	10	50	5.5	50th–58th	2
	10	100	7.1	58th	1
Spleen	10	50	5.9	27th–39th	5
	10	100	4.3	25th–55th	6
Heart	6	20	—	35th–42nd	4
	6	40	—	26th–41st	6
Kidney	6	20	—	27th–40th	6
	6	40	—	8th–30th	6

[1] Average weight, 20 gm.
[2] Daily injections, subcutaneously.

(6) Studies concerning the mechanism of action of the tissue extracts indicate that they prevented the formation of toxin by *S. aureus,* and also had some direct effect on toxin.

(7) Toxicity tests revealed that the brain and spleen extracts were relatively nontoxic, dosages equivalent to two percent of the body weight being well tolerated. Kidney and heart extracts were much more toxic, producing mortality in dosages as low as 0.3% of the body weight.

REFERENCES

BLAIR, J. E. 1939. The pathogenic staphylococci. Bacteriol. Rev. 3, 97–146.

CHAPMAN, G. H., BERENS, C., CURCIO, L., and NILSON, E. L. 1937A. The pathogenic *Staphylococcus:* Its isolation and differentiation from non-pathogenic types. J. Bacteriol. 33, 646.

CHAPMAN, G. H., BERENS, C., PETERS, A., and CURCIO, L. 1934. Coagulase and hemolysin tests as measures of the pathogenicity of the staphylococci. J. Bacteriol. 28, 343–363.

CHAPMAN, G. H., BERENS, C., NILSON, E. L., and CURCIO, L. G. 1938. The differentiation of pathogenic staphylococci from nonpathogenic types. J. Bacteriol. 35, 311–334.

CHAPMAN, G H., LIEB, C. W., BERENS, C., and CURCIO, L. 1937B. The isolation of probable pathogenic staphylococci. J. Bacteriol. 33, 533–543.

COWAN, S. T. 1938. Classification of staphylococci by precipitation and biological reactions. J. Pathol. 46, 31–45.

CRUICKSHANK, R. 1937. Staphylocoagulase. J. Pathol. Bacteriol. 45, 295–303.

DUDGEON, L. S., and SIMPSON, J. W. H. 1928. On the differentiation of the staphylococci, with special reference to the precipitin reactions. J. Hyg. (London) 27, 160–173.

HOLMAN, W. L. 1935. Studies on staphylococci. Am. J. Med. Sci. 189, 436–450.

PINNER, M., and VOLDRICH, M. 1932. Derivation of *Staphylococcus albus, citreus* and *roseus* from *Staphylococcus aureus.* J. Infect. Diseases 50, 185–202.

CHAPTER 4

Comparative Action of Probiotics from Beef Brain and of Penicillin on Staphylococcus Infections

PENICILLIN-SUSCEPTIBLE STRAINS OF *Staphylococcus aureus*

Carefully controlled clinical studies, together with the voluminous data amassed from widespread use of penicillin and the sulfonamides in various types of infections, have led to the search for and discovery of many other types of antibiotics. These all act through their toxic effects on the microorganisms.

Having established the fact that factors extracted from beef spleen, heart, kidney, and brain were effective both prophylactically and therapeutically against *Staphylococcus aureus* infections induced subcutaneously, intravenously, and intraperitoneally, experiments were undertaken to compare the newly discovered agents which *per se* are nonbactericidal, with a well-known antibiotic, penicillin.

Preliminary Studies

Forty-eight-hour broth cultures of a virulent strain of S. *aureus* No. 152, obtained from American Type Culture Collection, were used. The test animals, the BBC strain of mice, 3 to 6 months of age, were inoculated subcutaneously with 0.5 ml (1.5 LD$_{50}$) of the organism into the ventral abdominal region.

The brain extract, prepared as described previously (Chap. 1), was administered subcutaneously in the ventral abdominal region in doses of 50 mg daily. In the prophylactic experiments the first injection was given 2 hr before inoculation with the S. *aureus*. In the therapeutic experiments treatment was begun on the third day following inoculation with the infecting organism at which time there were typical suppurating lesions. The control animals received 0.25 ml of saline daily.

The penicillin was the commercial sodium salt manufactured in the Cheplin Laboratories. The dosage was 750, 1,000 and 2,000 Oxford units per day given subcutaneously in divided doses at 6-hr intervals in the ventral abdominal region. The procedure for inoculating the mice with the infecting organism was the same as that for the animals treated with brain extract. When the experiments were repeated, the injections of penicillin were given at 12-hr intervals. No difference was

34

observed in the response from that of animals treated at shorter intervals. The dosage levels were 5 to 10 times greater than the maximum amounts used by Robinson (1943) in the treatment of staphylococcic infections in mice.

In the first of the prophylactic series of experiments 40 mice were used, 10 serving as infected control animals, 10 receiving 50 mg of brain extract per day, and 2 groups of 10 each receiving penicillin in daily doses of 750 and 1,000 Oxford units, respectively. Daily treatments were continued until the lesions were healed as judged by the scabs dropping off and leaving the smooth new skin beneath.

When the experiment was repeated, a daily dose of 2,000 Oxford units of penicillin was substituted for the 750 Oxford-unit dose.

In the therapeutic experiments subcutaneous inoculations were made with 0.5 ml (1.5 LD_{50}) of the virulent 48-hr broth culture of S. aureus. Three days later, after the development of typical lesions, the animals were divided into four groups, each containing mice with infections of similar severity. One group of 10 served as infected untreated control animals and the other groups received, respectively, 50 mg of brain extract per day and 1,000 and 2,000 Oxford units of the sodium salt of penicillin per day in divided doses at 6-hr intervals until healing was complete. In the second experiment the doses of penicillin used were 750 and 1,000 Oxford units per day.

RESULTS

Prophylactic Experiments (Table 13)

All of the control mice developed suppurating lesions which were typical of staphylococcic infections in size and appearance. Of those animals which received the brain extract 2 hr before inoculations with the S. aureus, 80% developed needle-point lesions at the site of the injection and 20% developed lesions which were atypical, small, dry and nonsuppurating, and which healed within 4 to 9 days. In the animals treated with penicillin, 100% of those receiving 750 and 1,000 Oxford units per day and 80% of those receiving 2,000 Oxford units per day developed suppurating lesions which were smaller than those in the control animals but larger than the nonsuppurating lesions characteristic of the animals receiving the brain extract. As shown in Table 13, the average healing time for the groups of animals receiving penicillin was 13, 11, and 9 days, the interval being the shortest with the highest dosage of penicillin.

TABLE 13

COMPARISON OF THE PROPHYLACTIC ACTION OF BRAIN EXTRACT AND PENICILLIN ON SUBCUTANEOUS *Staphylococcus aureus* INFECTIONS IN MICE

Group	No. of Animals	Frequency and Type of Abscess	Mortality	Time of Healing, in Days, for Survivors	
		%	%	Range	Avg
Control	20	100 severe	90	(23)	23
Brain extract, 50 mg/day	20	80 needle point 20 moderate	0	(4–9)	7
Penicillin, 750 units/day	10	20 moderate 80 severe	70	(10–17)	13
Penicillin, 1,000 units/day	20	100 moderate	25	(8–16)	11
Penicillin, 2,000 units/day	10	20 none 80 moderate	10	(6–14)	9

Staphylococcus culture ATCC 152; dose used. 1.5 LD$_{50}$.

Therapeutic Experiments (Table 14)

In the animals treated with brain extract, the suppurating lesions typical of staphylococcic infections in mice apparently began to dry up as early as the second day following initiation of treatment. The lesions developed a dry, hemorrhagic appearance with the crust dropping off on the sixth to the ninth day. In the groups of animals receiving penicillin, suppuration continued for 3 to 9 days, with the first signs of healing appearing on the seventh day. None of the animals receiving the brain extract died. In the groups receiving penicillin the mortality was 80, 45 and 10%, the lowest mortality occurring in the animals receiving the highest dosage. On an average, healing required 23, 17, and 19 days in the survivors of the penicillin-treated animals.

TABLE 14

COMPARISON OF THE THERAPEUTIC ACTION OF BRAIN EXTRACT AND PENICILLIN ON SUBCUTANEOUS *Staphylococcus aureus* INFECTIONS IN MICE

Group	Number of Animals	Mortality	Average Time of Healing for Survivors
		%	Days
Control........................	20	95	27 (27)
Brain extract....................	20	0	7 (4–11)
Penicillin, 750 units/day.........	10	80	23 (21–26)
Penicillin, 1,000 units/day........	20	45	17 (11–19)
Penicillin, 2,000 units/day........	10	10	19 (18–22)

Staphylococcus culture, ATCC 152; dose used, 1.5 LD$_{50}$.

CONCLUSIONS

From the evidence presented it is apparent that brain extract, whether used as a prophylactic or as a therapeutic agent, is superior to penicillin in the dosages used for S. *aureus* infections under the conditions of these experiments.

PENICILLIN-RESISTANT STRAINS OF *Staphylococcus aureus*

Many investigators (Bondi and Dietz 1944A, 1944B; North and Christie 1945; Rammelkamp 1942; Rammelkamp and Maxon 1942; Robinson 1943; Spink and Ferris 1945A, 1945B; Spink and Hall 1945; Spink and Vivino 1944; Spink *et al.* 1944A, 1944B) have found that patients with staphylococcal infections do not always respond favorably to penicillin.

Having established the comparable effectiveness of probiotics from beef brain with penicillin on a strain of penicillin-susceptible *Staphylococcus aureus*, the present series of experiments was undertaken to determine if probiotics are likewise effective against penicillin-resistant strains. These studies included: (1) A comparison of the therapeutic and prophylactic effectiveness of brain extract and penicillin on subcutaneous infections induced by 24 pathogenic penicillin-resistant strains of S. *aureus*; and (2) a determination of any change in resistance of these organisms to brain extract on repeated exposure to the extract, as shown in *in vitro* and *in vivo* tests.

Experimental Work

The brain extract was prepared in batches from beef brain following the procedure described in Chap. 1. The various batches of extract were checked for effectiveness against a virulent strain of S. *aureus* (ATCC 152) which responded to penicillin therapy. The penicillin was the commercial sodium salt obtained from Abbott Laboratories, Schenley Laboratories, and the Cheplin Laboratories.

Twenty-four penicillin-resistant strains of organisms had been isolated from patients suffering from staphylococcic infections of various natures (chronic and acute osteomyelitis, empyema, axillary and retrobulbar abscesses and soft skin infections) in which penicillin therapy had been reported unsuccessful.[1] In some instances the or-

---

[1] We are indebted to Dr. C. H. Rammelkamp and Miss Marjorie Jewell of Evans Memorial Hospital, Boston; to Dr. W. W. Spink of the University of Minnesota; and to Dr. A. Bondi of Temple University, Philadelphia, for providing us with the 24 penicillin-resistant strains of S. *aureus*. Those obtained from Evans Memorial Hospital were: JR 8742, JB 9342, JB 81142, AP 10242, AP 10742, HH 11242, Ram. 10342, Ram. 92442, Ram. 91342, Ram. 10842, Ram. 87, Rosen 41, Merendale 515, Larabee 423, Nicolazzo 1124, Walbourne 411; those from Temple University were Bondi 446, and Bondi 161; and from the University of Minnesota, Rosen II CPF, Rosen III PF, Rosen I, Long III PF, Bernardo IIA, Bernardo II.

ganisms apparently had become resistant as a result of penicillin therapy since staphylococci isolated from these same lesions previous to treatment, had been sensitive to penicillin. All strains were maintained on blood agar slants until time of use.

Rockland Farm albino mice from 3 to 6 months of age were used in the *in vivo* tests.

Prophylactic Series

Control Animals.—For each of the 24 strains of *S. aureus* there was a control group of 6 infected, untreated animals. Saline suspensions of staphylococci were prepared with one loopful of a 24-hr nutrient broth culture of the organism per milliliter of saline. A uniform inoculum of 0.5 ml was maintained for all strains and injections made subcutaneously in the ventral abdominal region.

Experimental Animals.—An initial subcutaneous dose of 100 units of the sodium salt of penicillin in 0.1 ml of saline was given in the ventral abdominal region of mice in 24 groups of 6 animals each, 2 to 3 hr prior to subcutaneous infection with the staphylococci. Likewise 50 mg of brain extract was given subcutaneously to mice in each of the 24 groups of 6 animals each 2 to 3 hr prior to infection. The infecting dose of organisms was the same as that used for the control animals and daily treatment with 1,000 units of penicillin and with 50 mg of brain extract was given until death of the animal or until the lesions were healed as gauged by the dropping off of the scale leaving smooth new skin beneath.

Therapeutic Series

Each mouse in this series received subcutaneously in the ventral abdominal region 0.5 ml of a saline suspension of one loopful of a 24-hr culture of the organisms per milliliter. The animals were divided into control and experimental groups within 24 to 48 hr according to the degree of pathogenicity manifested. Animals showing similar degrees of reaction were distributed between the control and two experimental groups. For each of the 24 strains of staphylococci, 18 animals were used, 6 serving as infected untreated controls, 6 receiving penicillin, and 6 brain extract.

Control Animals.—As soon as the animals were divided into experimental groups they were given daily subcutaneous treatment with 1,000 units of penicillin or 50 mg of brain extract until the death of the animal or until the lesions healed completely.

RESULTS

Prophylactic Series (Table 15)

In the control animals of the prophylactic series the mortality ranged from 33⅓% with strain JB 9342 to 100% with 9 strains. Mortality for the total 144 control animals was 80% and occurred between the first and 24th days, one-half being dead by the fifth day (Fig. 4). Purulent lesions developed within 2 to 5 days and required 13 to 24 days (average, 19 days) for complete healing in the survivors. Abscess formation was followed by an extensive sloughing and the appearance of signs of listlessness, shaggy hair, cyanosis, and paralysis of the limbs.

Of the 144 animals treated with penicillin, 80% died within the first 17 experimental days, more than one-half being dead on the fifth day. In the individual groups, the mortality ranged from 33⅓% with 4 strains of organisms to 100% with 14 of the penicillin-resistant strains. All of the survivors in these groups of animals developed

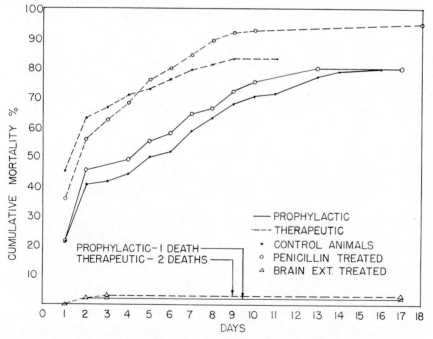

FIG. 4. CUMULATIVE MORTALITY IN A PROPHYLACTIC (432 MICE) AND A THERAPEUTIC (432 MICE) SERIES OF ANIMALS TESTING THE EFFECTIVENESS OF BRAIN EXTRACT AGAINST 24 PENICILLIN-RESISTANT STRAINS OF *Staphylococcus aureus*

purulent lesions averaging 18 days for healing with a range of 8 to 24 days.

Of the 144 animals receiving brain extract, one died of an injury; none died from the infection. Dry, scaly, nonsuppurating lesions, accompanied by severe sloughing in some cases, developed within 2 to 5 days in 86% of the group and these healed within 4 to 24 days (11 days average). There were no signs of toxic symptoms or paralysis among the brain-extract treated animals.

TABLE 15

COMPARATIVE RESPONSE OF MICE INFECTED WITH PENICILLIN-RESISTANT STRAINS (24) OF *S. aureus* TO PROPHYLACTIC AND THERAPEUTIC ADMINISTRATION OF PENICILLIN AND BRAIN EXTRACT

No. Animals	Treatment	% Mortality	Healing Time of Survivors in Days	
			Range	Avg
Prophylactic Series				
144	Control	80.0	(13–24)	19
144	Penicillin	80.0	(8–24)	18
144	Brain Extract	0.6	(4–24)	11
Therapeutic Series				
144	Control	84.0	(7–25)	18
144	Penicillin	95.0	(16–26)	22
144	Brain Extract	1.4	(3–17)	7

Eighteen mice were used for each penicillin-resistant strain of organisms: 6 control and 6 in each of the treated groups.

Inoculant 0.5 ml of a 24-hr nutrient broth culture, 1 loopful per ml.

In the therapeutic series, treatment consisted of 50 mg brain extract per day, 1000 units sodium salt of penicillin daily, while the controls received 0.3 ml saline daily.

In the prophylactic series both initial and subsequent doses were 50 mg of brain extract and 1000 units penicillin daily.

Therapeutic Series (Table 15)

In the group of 144 saline-injected control animals, mortality ranged from 66⅔% with 5 strains to 100% in 6 strains. Mortality for the entire group was 84%, more than one-half being dead on the third experimental day (Fig. 4). The purulent lesions of the survivors required from 7 to 25 days (average 18) for complete healing.

Of the 144 animals receiving penicillin, the total mortality was 95%, ranging from 83⅓% in 7 strains to 100% in 17 strains. More than one-half of the animals were dead on the third experimental day. The purulent lesions in the survivors required 16 to 26 days (average 22) for complete healing.

Of the 144 animals treated with brain extract two died: one (HH 11242) on the second, and one (Bondi 161) on the third experimental day. The healing time of the lesions of the 142 survivors ranged from 3 to 17 days with an average of 8 days.

Failure of Penicillin-resistant Strains of *Staphylococcus aureus* to become Resistant to Brain Extract, *in vitro* and *in vivo*

In Vitro.—For each of the 24 penicillin-resistant strains of staphylococci, 3 tubes were prepared containing 10 ml of nutrient broth and 0.2 ml veal infusion. One of these served as a control. To one was added 57.1 units of penicillin in the form of a freshly prepared 0.85% saline solution of the sodium salt of penicillin, containing 20 units per ml. To the third tube 100 mg of brain extract (100 mg per ml) was added. Each tube was inoculated with a standard loopful of a 24-hr nutrient broth culture of the organism and incubated at 37° C for 24 hr. Direct transfers were made every 24 hr (except for Sundays and holidays) to an identical series of 3 culture tubes. Twelve of the strains of organisms were thus treated for 37 days and the remaining 12 strains for 74 days. Visual determination of the turbidity was made each day.

In Vivo.—For each of the 24 penicillin-resistant strains of *S. aureus,* 3 test tubes containing nutrient broth media were inoculated with a standard loopful of a 24-hr culture of the organism. One of the tubes served as a control. To one experimental tube 57.1 units of penicillin in the form of sodium salt in saline (20 units per ml) was added, and to the other, brain extract (100 mg per ml) and all the tubes were incubated at 37° C. Transfers were made every three days. At the expiration of 12-hr, 15-day, and 30-day incubation periods, the potency of the cultures was determined by tests in animals. Rockland Farm albino mice, averaging 3 to 6 months of age, were inoculated subcutaneously with the organisms in the ventral abdominal region. The inoculum dosage for each strain was 0.5 ml of a 24-hr nutrient broth culture. Observations were made on the mortality and healing time of the lesions.

Results

In Vitro.—In Fig. 5 the turbidity readings selected for graphing were those for Tuesdays and Saturdays. Each point on the graph represents an average of the readings for the 12 strains on the specific days. The second series of 12 organisms (37-day experiment) was begun 2½ weeks after the completion of the first series of 12 (74-day experiment).

It is apparent that the overall turbidity readings of the second

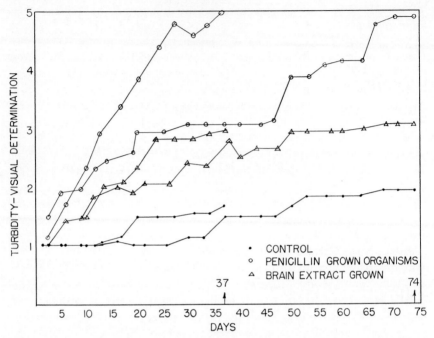

FIG. 5. AVERAGE TURBIDITY IN TWO SERIES OF PENICILLIN-RESISTANT STRAINS OF *Staphylococcus aureus*, 12 PER SERIES, CULTURED FOR 37 AND 74 DAYS, RESPECTIVELY, IN THE PRESENCE OF PENICILLIN AND OF BRAIN EXTRACT

Although it would appear from the graph that the organisms were stimulated only slightly less with brain extract than with penicillin, this is not an indication of the development of resistance in the case of the brain extract for its action is one of stimulation of growth with a concomitant conversion of the virulent organism to an avirulent form.

series are above those of the first series and it is felt that this apparent increase was due to the personal factor in visual determination. Within each series, however, the comparative control and experimental values probably are consistent.

Although it would appear from the graph that there is only a slight difference in the amount of stimulation of the growth of the microorganism by brain extract, as compared with penicillin, the action of these two materials is entirely different. Penicillin, when effective, acts by inhibiting growth, while the brain extract converts the yellow organism to a white variant with concomitant stimulation of growth *in vitro*.

It is apparent, therefore, that throughout the experimental periods (37 and 74 days) the organisms remained sensitive to the action of the brain extract, while in the presence of penicillin they retained their resistance to this antibiotic.

Twelve-hour Cultures *In Vivo*. (Table 16, Fig. 6) (432 Animals). —Total mortality in the control group was 82% and ranged from 33⅓% for 1 strain (Rosen I) to 100% for 12 strains; 71% died within 48 hr. For the animals receiving organisms from the penicillin-containing culture, the total mortality was 95% (range 66⅔% in one strain to 100% in 17 strains); 85% were dead within 2 days. Total mortality for the animals which received organisms grown for 12 hr in cultures containing brain extract was 2.8%. One died on the first day (Bernardo IIA), two on the third day (Nicolazzo 1124) and the last on the fourth day (Ram. 92442). No observations were made on the time required for healing of the lesions in the survivors of this group. One animal of the group which received Rosen IICPF organisms had a lesion in which there was suppuration for 2 days.

Fifteen-day Cultures (360 Animals).—The total mortality in the control series was 54% (range of 20% in Rosen 41 to 80% in 4 strains). The highest mortality occurred on the third day by which time 27% of the control animals were dead. The purulent lesions in the survivors required an average of 19 days for healing (range 10 to 32 days).

TABLE 16

COMPARATIVE MORTALITY IN MICE INFECTED WITH PENICILLIN-RESISTANT STRAINS (24) OF *Staphylococcus aureus* CULTURED 12 HR, 15 AND 30 DAYS IN A CONTROL MEDIUM AND IN MEDIA CONTAINING PENICILLIN AND BRAIN EXTRACT

No. Animals	Culture	% Mortality	Healing Time Survivors
	12-Hr Cultures		
			Days
144	Control	82.0	1
144	Penicillin	95.0	1
144	Brain extract	2.8	1
	15-Day Cultures		
120	Control	54.0	19 (10–32)
120	Penicillin	90.0	22 (9–30)
120	Brain extract	3.3	11 (4–23)
	30-Day Cultures		
120	Control	60.0	17 (4–29)
120	Penicillin	100.0	—
120	Brain extract	0.0	7 (4–16)

[1] No healing data recorded for test animals of 12-hr cultures.

18 mice were used for each strain of the penicillin-resistant organisms cultured for 12 hr; 15 mice for each strain cultured for 15 and 30 days; the animals were divided into 3 groups of equal number. Inoculant 0.5 ml, 1 loopful per ml.

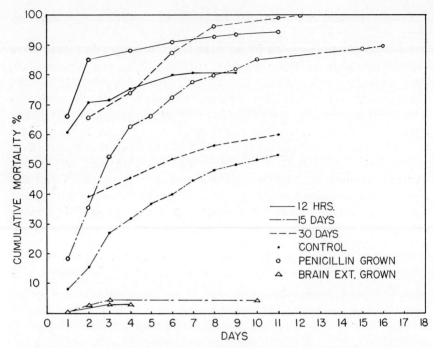

FIG. 6. CUMULATIVE MORTALITY IN MICE FOLLOWING INFECTION WITH PENICILLIN-RESISTANT *Staphylococcus aureus* ORGANISMS CULTURED FOR 12 HR (432 MICE), 15 DAYS (360 MICE) AND 30 DAYS (360 MICE) IN THE PRESENCE OF PENICILLIN AND OF BRAIN EXTRACT

The total mortality for the animals receiving organisms cultured for 15 days in the presence of penicillin was 90%, with a range of 60% for 4 strains to 100% for 16 strains; 53% were dead by the end of the third day. The lesions were purulent and required 22 days (range 9 to 30) for complete healing.

Of the 120 animals which received organisms cultured for 15 days with brain extract incorporated in the media, the total mortality was 3.3%, 1 animal dying on each of the first 3 days (Ram. 10842, Bondi 161, and Bernardo IIA), the fourth on the tenth day (Merendale 515). On the first day, all of the animals which received Bondi 161 had slightly suppurating lesions. One of these died and suppuration disappeared in two by the second day and in the remaining two by the fourth day. One animal of the group which received Rosen IICPF showed a slightly suppurative lesion on the second and third days. The healing time for the lesions was 11 days (range 4 to 23 days) in the animals of this group.

Thirty-day Cultures (360 Animals.)—Total mortality among the group of 120 control mice was 60%, ranging from 40% for 5 strains to 80% for 5 strains; 45% were dead by the fourth day. The average healing time for the purulent lesions in the survivors was 17 days with a range of 4 to 29 days.

Total mortality of the 120 animals, receiving organisms grown for 30 days in the presence of penicillin, was 100% within 12 days; 76% were dead by the fourth day.

There was no mortality among the 120 animals receiving organisms grown for 30 days in the presence of brain extract. The lesions which developed in 84% of the animals were nonsuppurating and required 4 to 16 days (or an average of 7 days) for complete healing. They were healed by the 11th day in 17 of the 24 groups of animals.

SUMMARY

Infections in mice with a series of 24 proven penicillin-resistant strains of *Staphylococcus aureus* responded to prophylactic and therapeutic administration of 80% alcohol-precipitated beef brain extract.

The turbidity studies on penicillin-resistant organisms, cultured in the continuous presence of brain extract for periods of 74 and 37 days, showed an increased growth as well as a conversion of the yellow S organism to a white R form, thus indicating that the organisms were sensitive to the extract throughout the experimental period. Similar studies with organisms which were cultured in the presence of penicillin demonstrated that the resistance to penicillin was maintained, as evidenced by increased turbidity. *In vivo* tests, after culture for 12 hr, 15 days, and 30 days, under these experimental conditions, demonstrated that the organisms became avirulent in the presence of the brain extract, and that this sensitivity to the extract was maintained throughout the experimental period.

REFERENCES

BONDI, A., and DIETZ, C. C. 1944A. Production of penicillinase by bacteria. Proc. Soc. Exptl. Biol. Med. *26*, 132–134.

BONDI, A., and DIETZ, C. C. 1944B. Relationship of penicillinase to the action of penicillin. Proc. Soc. Exptl. Biol. Med. *56*, 135–137.

NORTH, E. A., and CHRISTIE, R. 1945. Observations on the sensitivity of *Staphylococcus* to penicillin. Med. J. Australia, *32*, 44–46.

RAMMELKAMP, C. H. 1942. Resistance of *Staphylococcus aureus* to action of tyrothricin. Proc. Soc. Exptl. Biol. Med. *49*, 346–350.

RAMMELKAMP, C. H., and MAXON, T. 1942. Resistance of *Staphylococcus aureus* to the action of penicillin. Proc. Soc. Exptl. Biol. Med. *51*, 386–389.

ROBINSON, H. J. 1943. Toxicity and efficacy of penicillin. J. Pharmacol. 77, 70–79.

SPINK, W. W., and FERRIS, V. 1945A. Penicillin inhibitor from staphylococci which have developed resistance to penicillin in the human body. Proc. Soc. Exptl. Biol. Med. *59*, 188–190.

SPINK, W .W., and FERRIS, V. 1945B. Quantitative action of penicillin inhibitor from penicillin-resistant strains of staphylococci. Science *102*, 221–223.

SPINK, W. W., FERRIS, V., and VIVINO, J. J. 1944A. Comparative resistance *in vitro* of staphylococci to penicillin and to sodium sulfathiazole. Proc. Soc. Exptl. Biol. Med. *55*, 207–210.

SPINK, W. W., and HALL, W. H. 1945. Penicillin therapy at the University of Minnesota Hospitals. Ann. Internal Med. *22*, 510–525.

SPINK, W. W., and VIVINO, J. J. 1944. Sulfonamide-resistant staphylococci: correlation of *in vitro* sulfonamide-resistance with sulfonamide therapy. J. Clin. Invest. *23*, 267–278.

SPINK, W. W., WRIGHT, L. D., VIVINO, J. J., and SKEGGS, H. R. 1944B. p-Aminobenzoic acid production by staphylococci. J. Exptl. Med. 79, 331–339.

CHAPTER 5

Effects of Probiotics from a Variety of Tissues on a Number of Organisms

In addition to our in-depth studies of the effect of tissue extracts on *Staphylococcus aureus*, experiments were conducted (to a lesser degree) on other organisms. Included are a representative number of organisms of the colon-typhoid-dysentery groups and tubercle bacilli. Along with spleen and brain, fractions from a variety of tissues including heart, kidney, and liver also were used.

We have not attempted here to review the extensive literature on plant and animal tissues as sources of growth or "accessory" food factors and growth stimulants for bacteria. For information on this subject, the reader is referred to the work of Koser and Saunders (1938) Koser *et al.* (1936), and the excellent summary of Peskett (1933). It is, however, apparent in reviewing the literature that little is known regarding the mechanism of action of many of these substances. It is further apparent that none of the materials described possess the type of antibacterial action which has been exhibited by spleen and brain extracts.

IN VIVO STUDIES

Colon-Typhoid-Dysentery Group

Extracts from beef spleen, heart, brain, kidney, and liver were prepared in a manner identical with that previously described. After preparation of the extracts each was tested a minimum of 4 times for its effect on the following 6 organisms: *Escherichia coli, E. coli communior, Salmonella enteritidis, Eberthella typhosa, Bacillus paratyphosus A* and *Bacillus dysenteriae (Shigella)*. A series of three petri dishes, one serving as a control, the other two as experimental, were prepared for each organism. All 3 dishes contained 20 ml of nutrient agar, the experimental differing from the control in that one contained 0.5%, the other 1.0% dry weight of the extract to be tested. Each dish was inoculated with 0.1 ml of a saline-diluted (1 : 1,000,000) 24-hr culture of the organism. The dishes were swirled several times to ensure an equal distribution of the colonies. After

47

the dishes were incubated at 37° C for 48 hr the colonies were counted with the Wolffhuegel plate counter.

From these experiments it was clearly evident that the stimulatory material is not confined to spleen alone, but is found in other organs as well. Table 17, recording the stimulation of the six organisms by the different extracts in terms of percentage, is based directly on total plate counts. It will be noted from these results that heart and kidney extracts produce a greater percentage stimulation of growth than do brain, spleen, and liver extracts, the latter three being approximately equal in their stimulative power. It is to be noted, moreover, that one of the extracts (liver), with some organisms, undergoes a reversal in its activity if it is stored in the refrigerator. For example, the extract, when used before storage, showed stimulatory activity of 49% for *B. dysenteriae*, while after storage there was a depression of 100%.

Avirulent and Virulent Tubercle Bacilli

A number of investigators have observed that tissue extracts affect the growth of the tubercle bacillus. Arloing *et al.* (1937), testing the effect of glycerin extracts on the growth of the tubercle bacillus, found that extracts of kidney, liver, and spleen from normal guinea pigs retarded growth and that lung extracts enhanced it. Sarnowiec, (1939), employing glycerin extracts of tissues obtained from healthy and tuberculous guinea pigs and from rabbits, confirmed this but found no differences between the activity of tissues from infected and noninfected animals. Hirschberg and Arnold, (1938) using human tissue juices obtained by compression, were able to demonstrate that the heated and unheated juices of brain, heart, pancreas, liver, and kidney contained substances inhibitory for the organism. They postulated that the degree of inhibition of the individual juices is comparable to the resistance of that tissue against tuberculosis. The present investigations differ from the foregoing chiefly in the nature of the extract used which resulted from a different method of preparation.

In preliminary experiments, conducted on a nonquantitative basis, 2 types of media were employed: (1) 6% glycerin-agar, and (2) Long and Seibert's liquid synthetic medium. Two series of tubes, one containing glycerin-agar, the other the synthetic medium, were prepared and to them were added varying concentrations (0.5, 1.0, 2.0 and 5.0%) of each of the extracts. The terminal pH of the entire series was 7.2. The tubes containing liquid media were inoculated by

TABLE 17

PERCENTAGE GROWTH STIMULATION OF COLON-TYPHOID-DYSENTERY ORGANISMS SUBJECTED TO THE ACTION OF VARIOUS TISSUE EXTRACTS

Growth Response to 0.5 and 1% Extracts of

Organism	Heart		Kidney		Brain		Spleen		Liver Before Storage		Liver After Storage	
	0.5%	1.0%	0.5%	1.0%	0.5%	1.0%	0.5%	1.0%	0.5%	1.0%	0.5%	1.0%
E. coli............	171	466	8.6	115	18	59.3	15.7	21.3	23.6	23.9	21.9	10.0
E. coli communior......	228	425	54.0	116	29	52.0	34.0	43.6	2.6	2.6	−21.9	−53.6
S. enteritidis..........	225	440	48.0	87	36	70.0	18.0	38.0	58.0	49.0	1.6	−2.4
E. typhosa..........	325	606	45.0	124	47	97.0	44.1	76.0	31.3	12.1	−17.4	−38.0
B. paratyphosus A......	240	508	221.0	175	46	74.0	24.0	92.0	2.5	4.8	−9.8	−23.7
B. dysenteriae..........	157	386	94.0	151	48	103.0	49.6	39.7	58.0	49.0	−47.1	−63.7

floating a small flake of organisms on the surface; the glycerin-agar slants, by seeding with at least three pieces of growth. The incubation period at 37.5° C for the avirulent strain was 7 days, and for the virulent types 56 days. The tubes containing the latter were sealed with paraffin before incubation.

The test organisms were an avirulent strain of *M. tuberculosis* (American Type Culture Collection No. 607); an H37 strain (No. 8237) obtained from the same source; and strain G-2 and G-5 obtained from Dr. Guy P. Youmans of the Northwestern University Medical School. All of the organisms were grown on glycerin-agar for 28 days prior to their use in the experiments.

The results of these experiments are recorded in Table 18. It will be noted that all of the highest concentrations (5%) of the various organ extracts in either liquid or solid medium caused an apparent cessation of growth of the virulent organisms. Kidney and heart extracts, producing complete inhibition of growth at 2%, were apparently more effective than the other extracts. A marked difference between the response of the avirulent and virulent organisms to the various extracts was likewise apparent.

In order to determine whether the action of the organ extracts was bactericidal or bacteriostatic, the original inocula in all tubes of the H37 strain in which growth was suppressed were seeded upon glycerin-agar slants. Those organisms previously exposed to kidney, heart, brain, and liver extracts failed to grow, indicating bactericidal action for these extracts. The action of spleen extract, however, was apparently one of stasis, as organisms previously exposed to it grew profusely.

Since the preceding experiments, showing effects of tissue extracts on *M. tuberculosis*, had not been conducted on a quantitative basis, a culture technique was devised for a quantitative study of the effect of extracts of this nature. This technique, using a standard amount of inoculum, was an adaptation of the methods of Cooper and Cohn (1935) and of Youmans (1944). The surface-tension-reducing agent advocated by the former authors, and the emulsification procedure using an agate mortar and pestle, as described by Youmans, were omitted.

Ten milligrams of a 21-day-old culture of the organism grown on glycerin-agar slants were accurately weighed in a sterile test tube (Youmans, 1944). The culture was macerated for one minute by the stirring apparatus of Cooper and Cohn, and sterile medium added. The mixture was thoroughly shaken before the addition of sufficient

TABLE 18

EFFECT OF VARYING CONCENTRATIONS OF TISSUE EXTRACTS ON VIRULENT AND AVIRULENT TUBERCLE BACILLI

Strain	Avirulent M. tuberculosis ATCC 607		Virulent M. tuberculosis H-37—No. 8237		Virulent M. tuberculosis G-2 G-5	
Incubation	7 Days		56 Days		56 Days	
Extract Percent	6% Glycerin Agar	Long and Seibert's Medium	6% Glycerin Agar	Long and Seibert's Medium	Long and Seibert's Medium	
Control....	++++	++++	++++	++++	++++	++++
Brain						
0.5........	−	−	++++	+++	+++	+++
1.0........	−	−	+++	+	++	+
2.0........	−	−	+	−	+	−
5.0........	−	−	−	−	−	−
Kidney						
0.5........	+++	++++	+++	++	++	++
1.0........	+++	+++	+	−	−	+
2.0........	++	+++	−	−	−	−
5.0........	−	+++	−	−	−	−
Spleen						
0.5........	++++	++++	++++	++++	++++	++++
1.0........	+++	+++	++++	+++	+++	++
2.0........	+++	−	++++	++	++	++
5.0........	−	−	++	−	+	−
Heart						
0.5........	++++	++++	+++	++	++	++
1.0........	++++	++++	+	++	++	+
2.0........	+++	++	−	−	−	−
5.0........	+++	++	−	−	−	−
Liver						
0.5........	+++	++++	++++	++++	++++	++++
1.0........	++++	++++	++++	++++	++++	++++
2.0........	++++	++++	++++	++++	++++	++++
5.0........	++++	++++	−	−	−	−

++++ Good growth; +++ growth; ++slight growth; + very slight growth; − no growth.

medium to give a final concentration of 1 mg of organism per milliliter of solution (Youmans 1944). One-tenth milligram of the avirulent strain was seeded into control and experimental liquid media tubes prepared as in the previous experiments and placed in the incubator at 37.5° C for 7 days. One milligram of the virulent cultures was inoculated into a second series of tubes prepared in like manner and incubated for 21 days. All cultures were shaken after 3 and 5 days.

At the end of the incubation period the weight of the organisms was obtained by a filtration method involving the use of alundum crucibles of fine porosity. The organisms were filtered in the weighed crucibles and boiling distilled water was poured through several times. The crucibles were then dried and reweighed.

The results, presented in Table 19, are similar in most respects to those in the preliminary investigations. It is of particular interest that kidney extract, which was one of the best inhibitors of growth for the virulent strains, was the best stimulator for growth of the avirulent organism.

IN VIVO STUDIES ON SALMONELLA WITH PROBIOTICS FROM BEEF BRAIN

Experimental Animals Used in in Vivo Studies

The experimental animals used in the study of crude probiotics on *Salmonella typhi* were a strain of white Swiss albino mice procured from the Texas Inbred Mice Co. Both sexes were used and are designated in the procedure of the experiments. The animals ranged in age from 10 to 14 weeks. These animals are highly susceptible to relatively small numbers of the *Salmonella*. Virulence of the organism was based on its ability to kill its host.

Selection of Suitable Media for the Growth of the Organism

Although *Salmonella typhi* is not considered a fastidious organism, considerable difficulty was at first encountered in culturing the organism from the lyophilized state. Finally, after trying a variety of media, a suitable procedure was attained which allowed growth of an optimal virulent nature. A light inoculum was placed on chorioallantoic membrane of a 10-day-old chick embryo. Excellent growth was obtained in 24 hr. From this, a loopful was removed and transferred to a slant containing Trypticase Soy Agar. This medium, which is a general-purpose medium containing trypticase, phytone, NaCl, and agar, appeared to enhance the growth of the organism better than the other media tested.

Preservation of the Organism

Since the culture of the organism obtained from American Type Culture Co. was lyophilized it was not necessary to prepare any additional amount for a stock culture. As is well-known, a culture prepared in this way can be stored under refrigeration for periods exceeding one year. In our experience reconstitution is best achieved by the method previously described, i.e., depositing a few flakes of the lyophilized culture on the chorioallantoic membrane of a chick embryo.

Determination of Salmonella Dosage in Mice (LD$_{50}$)

The following is a brief discussion of the procedure used for the preparation of the bacterial suspension and the determination of the LD$_{50}$.

TABLE 19

QUANTITATIVE EFFECTS OF TISSUE EXTRACTS ON GROWTH OF TUBERCLE BACILLI USING A STANDARD INOCULUM

Organism	Avirulent ATCC No. 607		Virulent H37		Virulent G-2		Virulent G-5	
Extract %	Growth	Yield Mg	Growth	Yield Mg	Growth	Yield Mg	Growth	Yield Mg
Control	++++P[1]	17.7	++++P	4.5	++++P	3.4	++++P	2.1
Brain								
0.5	++++P	24.2	++++P	5.5	+++	2.7	+++	1.5
1.0	—	—	++++P	4.2	+++	1.8	++	0.2
2.0	—	—	++++P	3.6	++	1.1	—	0.1
5.0	—	—	++++P	2.9	++	0.9	—	—
Kidney								
0.5	++++P	46.7	++	1.3	++	2.2	++	1.0
1.0	+++++P	42.0	+++	1.1	++	1.2	+++	0.8
2.0	++++P	94.0	++	0.7	+++	0.9	+++	0.3
5.0	+++	96.0	—	0.1	—	0.2	++	0.2
Spleen								
0.5	+++P	86.0	++++P	4.8	++++P	3.3	+++P	2.1
1.0	++	24.0	+++	4.0	++++	2.3	+++P	1.8
2.0	—	—	+++	2.3	++++	2.0	+++	1.0
5.0	—	—	++	1.3	+++	0.9	++	0.4
Heart								
0.5	++++P	73.1	++++P	4.6	++++	2.8	+++P	2.3
1.0	++	58.1	+++	1.8	+++	1.1	+++P	2.0
2.0	—	—	++	0.2	+++	0.3	+++	0.5
5.0	—	—	—	—	++	0.1	+++	0.1
Liver								
0.5	++++P	68.0	++++P	3.3	++	2.6	+++P	2.2
1.0	+++++P	50.0	+++	1.8	+++	1.4	++	1.1
2.0	+++++P	36.0	+++	1.2	+++	1.1	—	0.5
5.0	++++	30.6	++	0.7	++	0.5	—	0.2

[1] P Pellicle or surface growth; ++++ good growth; +++ growth; ++ slight growth; + very slight growth; — no growth.

Trypticase Soy Agar slants were inoculated with the mother culture of *Salmonella typhi* 24 hr prior to the challenge date. Upon removal of the slants after 24 hr of incubation, five milliliters of Tyrode solution (Difco) plus 4–5 glass beads were added to the tubes. The growth on the slant was then removed by slow agitation of the tube. The heavy suspension was placed in a volumetric flask and diluted with Tyrode solution. Different density suspensions were prepared by this method and the densities of the various suspensions were adjusted on a nephelometer. Light transmission readings were used as a measure of the density of suspensions. These different suspensions were then inoculated intraperitoneally at various dosage levels into groups of mice, ten animals per group. Observations on the condition of the infected animals were made every 24 hr for one week. It was found that transmission readings of 96% or less resulted in 100% mortality and that a light transmission reading of 98.5% represented the LD_{50} and corresponded to a dose of approximately 250,000 organisms.

Preparation of a Semipurified Synthetic Mouse Diet

From the results of other investigators and from our preliminary investigations on *Salmonella* infection in mice, it was decided that a controllable synthetic and semipurified diet should be employed in all of our experiments dealing with this infection. The formula for the diet which was finally adopted was derived from that developed by J. Milton Bell (1962) and modified by the addition of 2.5% gum arabic and 5% talc powder to allow pelleting the mixture. Its composition is given in the accompanying Table 20.

Preparation of Crude Brain Extract

Since this organism (*Salmonella typhi*) had not been employed to any great extent in previous brain extract studies, preliminary experiments were performed using only the crude alcoholic extract, in order to evaluate its effectiveness as a protective agent.

Fresh beef brains were obtained from a local abattoir, the capsular material removed and the brain material washed free of blood. The cleansed brains were then ground in a meat grinder, weighed, and distilled water added to the mass in equal proportion (weight by volume). The mixture was refrigerated for a period of 24 hr, then centrifuged at 2000 rpm for 20 min, and the supernatant liquid decanted. Enough 95% alcohol was added to the supernatant to produce a final alcoholic concentration of 80%. This mixture was allowed to stand at room temperature and then filtered through Whatman No.

TABLE 20

BELL'S SEMIPURIFIED SYNTHETIC MOUSE DIET

Ingredient	Per 100 Gm of Diet
Part I	
Casein, vitamin-free, gm	22.3
Cornstarch, gm	44.3
Sucrose, gm	11.2
Salt mixture[1], gm	6
Cellulose, gm	11.2
Corn oil, gm	5
Part II	
Menadione, mg	10
Choline, mg	135
Thiamine, mg	0.3
Riboflavin, mg	0.4
Niacin, mg	0.3
Pyridoxine, mg	0.1
Pantothenic acid, mg	0.9
Folic acid, mg	2.5
Biotin, mg	0.01
Vitamin A, stabilized, IU	50.0
Vitamin B12, μg	0.5
Vitamin D, IU	20.0
Inositol, mg	0.1
p-aminobenzoic acid, mg	1.2

[1] Salt mixture composed of $CaHPO_4 \cdot 2H_2O$, 25.1; $CaCO_3$, 42.1; NaCl, 22.4; KCl, 6.69; $FeSO_4 \cdot 7H_2O$, 18; $MgSO_4 \cdot 5H_2O$, 0.05; and KI calcium stearate, 0.01%.

1 filter paper. The supernatant portion was distilled to remove the alcohol and the remaining mixture was brought to wet-dryness on a steam bath. The substance was reconstituted with distilled water, the pH adjusted to 7.0, Seitz filtered, dry weight determined, and bottled for testing.

In Vivo Experiments

For the most part the *in vivo* results which are reported are based on prophylactic treatments. In this procedure the experimental animals were given a subcutaneous injection of the test preparation in the ventral abdominal region daily for five successive days. In a few experiments animals were treated by oral administration, in which case the test material was given twice daily for five successive days. On the fifth day following the last injection of test material, all experimental animals (in addition to a control group of animals) were inoculated intraperitoneally with an LD_{50} dose of *Salmonella* organisms.

A limited number of assays were performed involving therapeutic treatment. In 1 procedure the test material was injected 2 to 4 hr following injection of the organism, and then repeated injections were made every 24 hr for a period of 2 days; the other, a combined prophylactic-therapeutic procedure, involved injections of the test material 5 days prior to and 5 days following injection with the *Salmonella* organism.

The first experiments on *Salmonella* in mice were restricted to the effect of crude brain extract and included those conducted before the adoption of a semipurified synthetic mouse diet. The results are based on prophylactic and therapeutic formats of treatments administered subcutaneously and orally. The dosage of crude brain extract varied with the route of inoculation. In case of subcutaneous treatment, each experimental animal received 20 mg per day for 2 days in the therapeutic series. In the case of oral administration, each experimental animal received 25 mg twice daily for 5 days, using the prophylactic procedure.

Results of *in Vivo* Experiments.—The results of these preliminary investigations are given in Tables 21, 22, and 23.

Earlier experiments with animals treated with crude brain extract, which were conducted in an attempt to induce protection against

TABLE 21

EFFECT OF BRAIN EXTRACT ON *Salmonella* INFECTION IN MICE

Prophylactic Series—Crude Brain Subcutaneous Treatment

Sex	No. of Animals per Group Exptl.	Control	% Mortality Exptl.	Control
Females	10	10	10	30
Females	10	10	70	80
Males	7	7	29	57
Males	10	10	30	80
Females	10	10	10	40
Females	20	20	15	40
Females	7	7	71	100
Males	10	10	0	40
Females	10	10	0	30
Males	10	10	0	30
Total	104	104	20	50

TABLE 22

EFFECT OF BRAIN EXTRACT ON *Salmonella* INFECTION IN MICE

Therapeutic Series—Crude Brain Subcutaneous Treatment

Sex	No. of Animals per Group Exptl.	Control	% Mortality Exptl.	Control
Females	10	10	20	30
Females	20	20	35	40
Males	10	10	40	40
Total	40	40	32.5	37.5

TABLE 23
EFFECT OF BRAIN EXTRACT ON *Salmonella* INFECTION IN MICE

Prophylactic Series—Crude Brain Oral Treatment

| Sex | No. of Animals per Group | | % Mortality | |
	Exptl.	Control	Exptl.	Control
Females	8	10	12.5	30
Females	10	10	90	80
Males	11	10	54.5	80
Females	11	10	36.3	40
Total	40	40	50	57.5

artificially-induced *Salmonella* infection, yielded inconsistent results. For this reason experiments were designed to determine whether these inconsistencies could be eliminated by employing animals raised on the semipurified synthetic diet (Table 20).

The results are based on prophylactic treatments. Each experimental animal received subcutaneous injections of 20 mg of crude brain extract daily for 5 days. All animals were challenged within 2 hr after the fifth treatment. The results of this study are recorded in Table 24.

TABLE 24
EFFECT OF BRAIN EXTRACT ON *Salmonella* INFECTION IN MICE

Prophylactic Series—Crude Brain Treatment—Animals
Raised on Semipurified Synthetic Diet

| Sex | No. of Animals per Group | | % Mortality | |
	Exptl.	Control	Exptl.	Control
Males	10	10	0	50
Males	10	10	0	40
Females	10	10	20	80
Females	10	10	0	40
Females	10	10	10	50
Females	10	10	10	60
Females	10	10	20	70
Total	70	70	8.9	55.7

In these experiments the observation was made that the mortalities which occurred in the control groups and in the experimental groups appeared after 24 to 48 hr. Because of this it was felt that therapeutic treatment combined with prophylactic might be effective in reducing the mortality which occurred 24 to 48 hr after cessation of treatment. Consequently, experiments were conducted in which experimental animals, after receiving subcutaneous injections of 20 mg crude brain extract daily for 5 days, and being challenged with an LD_{50} dose of *Salmonella*, were treated 24 and 48 hr later with additional subcutaneous

TABLE 25

EFFECT OF BRAIN EXTRACT ON *Salmonella* INFECTION IN MICE

Combined Prophylactic-Therapeutic Series—Crude Brain Subcutaneous
Treatment—Animals Raised on Semipurified Synthetic Diet

| | No. of Animals per Group | | % Mortality | |
Sex	Exptl.	Control	Exptl.	Control
Males	10	10	0	50
Males	10	10	0	60
Females	10	10	0	80
Females	10	10	0	50

injections of 20 mg crude brain extract. The results of this study are recorded in Table 25.

CONCLUSIONS

From the above results it may be concluded that: (1) Swiss albino mice exhibit a definite increase in susceptibility to induced *Salmonella* infection when raised on a semipurified synthetic diet; (2) animals raised on a semipurified synthetic diet, when treated on a combined prophylactic-therapeutic basis with crude brain extract, exhibit complete protection against induced *Salmonella* infection.

REFERENCES

ARLOING, F., THEVENOT, L., and VIALLIER, J. 1937. Influence of extracts of various organs on homogenous liquid cultures of human tubercle bacillus. Compt. Rend. Soc. Biol. *124*, 164–165.

BELL, J. M. 1962. Nutrient requirements of the laboratory mouse. Natl. Acad. Sci.-Natl. Res. Council, Publ. *990*.

COOPER, H. J., and COHN, M. L. 1935. A mechanical device for preparing fine suspensions of tubercle bacilli and other microorganisms. J. Lab. Clin. Med. *21*, 428–431.

HIRSCHBERG, N., and ARNOLD, L. 1938. The effect of human tissue juices on tubercle bacilli. Am. Rev. Tuberc. 37, 598–611.

KOSER, S. A., and SAUNDERS, F. 1938. Accessory growth factors for bacteria and related microorganisms. Bacteriol. Rev. *2*, 99–160.

KOSER, S. A., SAUNDERS, F., FINKLE, I. J., and SPOELSTRA, R. C. 1936. Bacterial nutrition. II. Distribution of a growth-stimulating factor in animal and plant tissues. J. Infect. Diseases 58, 121–127.

PESKETT, G. L. 1933. Growth factors of lower organisms. Biol. Rev., Cambridge Phil. Soc. *8*, 1–24.

SARNOWIEC, W. 1939. The influence of culture filtrates from different bacteria on the growth of tubercle bacilli in deep cultures. Zentr. Bakt. Parasitenk. *143*, 232–233.

YOUMANS, G. P. 1944. An improved method for testing of bacteriostatic agents using virulent human-type tubercle bacilli. Proc. Soc. Exptl. Biol. Med. *57*, 119–122.

CHAPTER 6

The Effect of Probiotics from Beef Brain on Encephalomyocarditis Virus in Mice

To broaden the scope of the investigations of the effects of probiotics, a limited number of experiments were conducted on viral infections. The MM strain selected for our initial studies was isolated first by Jungeblut and Dalldorf (1943) from a hamster brain inoculated with material from human spinal cord and medulla taken from a patient who had died of clinically diagnosed paralytic disease.

All of the experiments undertaken in this study were conducted (excepting for minor details) in an identical manner. The procedure consisted essentially of a comparison of symptom development and mortality in control and experimental mice infected with the encephalomyelitis virus (MM). All mice were infected via the foot pad route. The experimental animals were treated both prophylactically and therapeutically with extracts of beef brain.

Two series of experiments were performed. In the first series, Rockland All-Purpose strain mice were used, and in the second series Swiss albino mice.

SERIES I—MATERIALS AND METHOD

The mice were the Rockland All-Purpose strain and approximately 28 days of age. The water-soluble alcoholic extract of beef brain used in these experiments was prepared as described in Chap. 1. The virus employed (MM), although secured from two different sources, showed no appreciable difference in Minimal Infective Dose (MID).

Preparation of Virus

The virus, originally obtained from a frozen saline suspension, was inoculated at a dosage of 0.04 ml into 10 mice. At the end of 3 days the mice were sacrificed and a 10% saline suspension of virus prepared from their pooled brains. This material and suspension similarly prepared from time to time were stored in the frozen state for use in the experiments. Prior to use, however, the Minimal Infective Dose (MID), defined as that amount of virus which would paralyze or kill 50% of the animals in 10 days, was determined for the 10% suspensions of pooled virus. This was done by inoculating groups of 10 mice each

59

with 0.03 ml of the virus suspension of dilutions ranging from 10^{-6} to 10^{-10}. Ten times the MID was used in the experiments, and this dose was rechecked at the middle and again at the end of the experiment.

In Vivo Experiments

In the first experiment 100 animals were used, 50 serving as experimental and 50 as control. The experimental animals were given subcutaneous injections of 100 mg of the water-soluble alcoholic extract of beef brain for a period of 35 days, and on the sixth day received 0.03 ml of a 10^{-8} (MID 10^{-9}) dilution of a 10% suspension of the virus (MM) via the foot pad. The 50 control animals were observed for the same period of time (35 days) and received the same amount of virus on the same day and by the same route as the experimentals, but received no brain extract.

RESULTS

The results of this experiment are recorded in Experiment 1, of Table 26. It is to be noted that in both groups of animals, a certain number were discarded in estimating our figures for frequency of symptoms and total mortality. In the control group the 6 animals which were rejected were those dying within 48 hr after inoculation with the virus, or dying without symptoms of infection at a later date. The same is true for the eight rejects in the experimental group but, in addition, animals dying prior to inoculation with the virus were discarded. On the basis of the remaining 44 control animals and 42 experimentals, it is apparent that the brain extract affords marked protection over the control group, against such observed symptoms as rapid breathing, eye edema, staring-fixed look, tremor, spinning, arched back, flattened posterior, and paralysis. Protection against mortality was equally significant. No deaths occurred in the experimental group later than seven days following inoculation with the virus, while control animals continued to die for 24 days. The peak mortality of six days was the same for both groups.

Because of evidence of moderate toxicity of brain extract at the dosage used in the foregoing experiment, a second experiment was conducted in which the daily dosage of the extract was lowered, injections of 25 and 50 mg being given on alternate days. With this exception, and also the fact that a larger number of animals (150) equally divided into controls and experimentals, were used, the experiment was conducted the same as Experiment 1.

It was not necessary to discard any animal from this experiment for the reasons given in the first experiment; consequently, the figures for symptom development and mortality in the control and experimental animals are based on a total of 75 animals in each group (Table 26, Experiment 2). The lower dosage of extract used in Experiment 2, while affording protection, is evidently less effective than the higher dosage used in Experiment 1. Moreover, the experimental animals continued to die for a period of 12 days after virus inoculation as compared to seven days in Experiment 1. There was a slight shift in mortality, however, the controls peaking at six days, the experimental at eight.

In a third experiment, the number of animals was reduced to 25 each for both the control and experimental groups. In addition, although the total period of observation was the same as that for Experiments 1 and 2, the experimental animals received their combined prophylactic and therapeutic treatment with brain extract over a period of only 15 days at a dosage of 25 mg per day. This was done because it was felt that the prolongation of mortality after virus inoculation in the experimental animals in Experiment 2, as compared with Experiment 1, might have been due in some measure to a cumulative toxic effect of the extract. The remainder of the procedure was unaltered.

The results of this experiment, shown in Table 26, Experiment 3, were somewhat better than in Experiment 2, both as to number of animals developing symptoms and total mortality. The degree of protection was also somewhat better, and the mortality range was confined to a period of five days. Peak mortality in the controls was five days as against seven in the experimental.

The results of these three experiments are typical of a large number which have been performed. Among them are experiments in which the extract has been used successfully solely as a prophylactic or solely as a therapeutic agent.

The experiments were repeated using another strain of mice and administering the probiotics orally as well as by injection.

SERIES II—MATERIALS AND METHOD

The experimental animals were the moderately inbred Swiss albino strain of mice. When referring to the virulence of the virus in these experiments, the mortality of the test animals was used as the criterion. The virulence of the virus employed, which was dependent on the age of the experimental animal, reached its highest degree and consistency

TABLE 26

EFFECTS OF COMBINED PROPHYLACTIC AND THERAPEUTIC ADMINISTRATION OF BRAIN EXTRACT ON (MM) VIRUS INFECTION IN MICE

Animal Groups	No. of Animals	Days Treated	Dosage per Day	% Animals Developing Symptoms	Total Mortality No. Animals	%	Days Before Death Range
			Experiment 1				
Control	44[1]	—	—	89	39	89	4–24
Experimental	42[1]	35	100 mg	11	9	11	5–7
			Experiment 2				
Control	75	—	—	57	43	57	4–18
Experimental	75	35	25–50 mg	28	19	25	5–12
			Experiment 3				
Control	25	—	—	64	16	64	4–13
Experimental	25	15	25 mg	28	6	24	6–10

[1] Of the original 50 animals in each group, 6 controls and 8 experimentals were rejected. *See* Text.

with animals ranging in age from 3 to 4 weeks. Animals of this age group were used in the following experiments.

Preparation of Virus Particles

The initial stock virus suspension was obtained from the Wm. S. Merrell Co. Based on an intraperitoneal inoculation of 0.25 ml, it had an LD_{50} (in young mice) of $10^{-8.3}$. The preparation of the stock virus "pool" was as follows: 20 Swiss female mice, ranging in weight from 9 to 14 gm, were inoculated intracerebrally with 0.03 ml of a 10^{-4} dilution of the stock suspension. After 40 to 49 hr the brains of the surviving 18 mice were removed aseptically and placed in a sterile beaker. Two ml of a 50% rabbit serum-saline mixture was added for each brain, or a total of 36 ml and suspension obtained with a Waring blender. The resulting 10% suspension was divided into 1-ml portions, placed in glass ampoules and sealed. In order to retain virulence of the virus the ampoules were stored at $-72°$ C. By this method of storage the virus was found to retain complete virulence for a period of not less than 2 yr.

Experimental Infection

In preliminary experiments, it was established that mice of all ages die following inoculation by any of the usual routes with a 10^{-7} dilution of a suspension of viral infected brain tissue from moribund mice. Within 72 or 96 hr such inoculations produce symptoms of ruffled fur, lethargy and flaccid paralysis, the hind legs being affected first. These symptoms are usually followed by prostration and death.

Determination of Virus Dosages

Virus suspensions were prepared from the mother stock by serial dilution with physiological saline. The prepared dilutions, ranging from $10^{-7.5}$ to 10^{-9}, were tested by intraperitoneal injection of 0.25 ml per mouse. The LD_{50} was found to be $10^{-8.2}$ and was used in all experiments employing this virus.

In Vivo Experiments

In the prophylactic experiments the test material was administered orally or by subcutaneous injection daily for five successive days. One to three hours after the last injection of the test material, all experimental animals, in addition to the control group, were inoculated intraperitoneally with an LD_{50} dose of EMC virus.

A small number of *in vivo* assays were performed using a therapeutic format of inoculation. This assay involved injection of the test material one to two hours following the injection of the virus and then repeated injections every 24 hr for a period of 5 days.

Subcutaneously treated animals received a dry weight inoculum of 20 mg per day, while orally treated animals received a dry weight inoculum of 25 mg twice daily.

RESULTS

The results of the prophylactic series of experiments using Swiss albino mice in which the animals were treated by subcutaneous injection, are given in Table 27. They compare favorably with those in which the Rockland strain was used.

TABLE 27

PROPHYLACTIC SERIES—CRUDE BRAIN SUBCUTANEOUS TREATMENT

| | No. of Animals per Group | | % Mortality | |
	Exptl.	Control	Exptl.	Control
	10	10	30	80
	10	10	10	40
	10	10	10	50
	10	10	10	60
	10	10	0	40
Total	50	50	12	54

When the brain extract was administered orally the results, as may be seen from Table 28, are negative. The results of the therapeutic series, in which the extract was administered both subcutaneously (Table 29), and orally (Table 30), showed questionable, if any, improvement. Further experiments are necessary to determine if higher dosages might be effective.

SUMMARY

The only treatment resulting in significant improvement was that in which animals received crude brain extract subcutaneously on a prophylactic basis. The protection obtained in this case was significant in being not only consistent with, but substantially higher than that obtained in our earlier investigations when the experimental animals were treated at the same dosage level of crude brain extract.

TABLE 28

PROPHYLACTIC SERIES—CRUDE BRAIN ORAL TREATMENT

| No. of Animals per Group | | % Mortality | |
Exptl.	Control	Exptl.	Control
12	10	41.6	40
8	10	37.5	80
10	10	50	70
10	10	50	50

TABLE 29

THERAPEUTIC SERIES—CRUDE BRAIN SUBCUTANEOUS TREATMENT

| No. of Animals per Group | | % Mortality | |
Exptl.	Control	Exptl.	Control
10	10	40	30
10	10	40	50
10	10	60	50
20	20	45	45

TABLE 30

THERAPEUTIC SERIES—CRUDE BRAIN ORAL TREATMENT

| No. of Animals per Group | | % Mortality | |
Exptl.	Control	Exptl.	Control
10	10	30	30
10	10	30	70
10	10	40	50
—	—	—	—
Total 30	30	33.3	50

REFERENCE

JUNGEBLUT, C. W., and DALLDORF, G. 1943. Epidemiological and experimental observations on the possible significance of rodents in a suburban epidemic of poliomyelitis. Am. J. Public Health 33, 169–172.

CHAPTER 7

Importance of Diet and Strain in Assay of Probiotics

In our early researches it was possible to produce local staphylococcal infections in mice by the intracutaneous injection of 100,000 organisms. The majority of mice treated with such a limited number of organisms would recover.

The LD_{50} for mice of this same strain of staphylococci was in the neighborhood of 500,000 organisms. The animals so treated would survive for an average of approximately five days, with death following more rapidly with higher doses. As time progressed, the virulence of the strain seemed to decrease, larger and larger doses being required to produce death in the same strain of mice. Furthermore, in the later experiments, when a minimal lethal dose was administered, the animals would die within 24 hr; whereas, in the early researches, under similar conditions, the animals would survive for approximately 8 to 10 days.

Accepted methods of enhancing virulence, such as cultivation on selective or enriched media [(SA-110) (Chapman 1946) and brain heart infusion broth] or cultivation under increased CO_2 tension failed to produce any noticeable change in the lethality of the organism for the test animals used. A thorough study was made of the effect of such variables as age and sex of the animals.

In female mice there was no appreciable change in mortality in the age range of 4 to 26 weeks. Beyond this age the animals appeared slightly more susceptible to infection. With male animals it was difficult to determine the effect of age on the course of the infection since beyond ages 12 to 13 weeks the mortality was influenced by fighting and secondary infections in the animals. In all experiments, both for males and females, an attempt was made to keep the age limit below 12 weeks.

Strains of *Staphylococcus aureus* were isolated from human lesions and many strains obtained from other laboratories but little variation was found in the virulence of the different strains. The possibility exists that all of the strains which had been tested had changed as a result of exposure to antibiotics which had become so widely used. Also, there remained the possibility that it was not the organisms which had changed, but the animals or the diet. Inasmuch as commercial diets frequently contain a percentage of animal organs which can be

66

a source of crude probiotics, it occurred to us that the commercial diet which we were using might be the seat of our difficulties.

With these thoughts in mind an investigation into the importance of strain and diet was undertaken.

MATERIALS AND METHODS

Culture

A single strain of S. *aureus*, designated in our laboratories "Original Strain," was used throughout the series of experiments. This organism had its origin in a human infection of the tonsil. It fermented mannitol, was coagulase-positive, and showed resistance to pencillin as well as to a number of other antibiotics. It was maintained in the lyophilized state and was cultured for use in Difco SA-110 medium. Only three subcultures from the mother culture on SA-110 medium were made, another mother culture being prepared at the end of this time from a fresh tube of the lyophilized organism.

Mice

Four strains of mice were employed in these experiments: Boontucky, Swiss albino, C3H/HeJ, and C57B1. The Boontucky strain, originally derived from the Rockland All-Purpose strain of mouse, has been maintained through random breeding in our laboratories over a period of years. The Swiss albino is a moderately inbred strain procured from Texas Inbred Mice Co. The C3H/HeJ and the C57B1 are highly inbred strains procured from the Jackson Memorial Laboratories.

Inoculum

Organism inoculum for all experiments was prepared in the following manner. A culture grown aerobically on SA-110 medium for 24 hr at 37.5° C was washed with sterile 0.85% NaCl to remove all of the organisms. The suspension of organisms was then placed in a volumetric flask and shaken vigorously to break up clumping and to ensure uniform dispersion. Samples of the suspension were removed and diluted with physiological saline to give predetermined transmission levels on a nephelometer. The transmission readings on the scale of the instrument, which are a measure of the density of suspensions, were correlated with bacterial counts (Table 31). Each level of organism suspension to be tested was then inoculated subcutaneously at a dosage of 0.5 ml in the ventral groin region of the animals.

TABLE 31

CORRELATION OF BACTERIAL COUNTS WITH PERCENT LIGHT
TRANSMISSION READINGS OF STAPHYLOCOCCAL SUSPENSIONS

% Transmission Reading	Bacterial Count per 0.5 Ml
30	25×10^8
40	10×10^8
50	60×10^7
60	32×10^7
70	22×10^7
80	15×10^7
90	12×10^7

Diet

In the experiments on genetic strain difference, all animals were maintained on the commercial Rockland Mouse Diet. In the experiments relating to diet and virulence, the control animals were maintained on the Rockland Diet. The experimental animals were fed on a diet of the following composition: corn, 83.15%; casein, 16.0%; DL-methionine, 0.85%. In previous experiments this diet had been found adequate for growth requirements of mice (Healy 1957).

RESULTS

In dietary experiments, the Boontucky strain only was investigated. Mice of both sexes, ranging in age from 9 to 11 weeks, and in weight from 25 to 30 gm, were used. The experimental mice were kept on the "Special Diet" for a period of 6 to 8 weeks before comparing their infectivity by S. aureus with that for mice fed the commercial Rockland Mouse Diet.

The results are illustrated in Fig. 7 which is a composite of a number of experiments conducted. From this illustration it can be ascertained that the susceptibility of mice to staphylococcal infection is closely associated with diet and can be greatly modified by alteration in this factor. In the case of the experimental mice, a transmission level of 60% (32×10^7 organisms) was sufficient to produce 100% mortality; whereas, in the control animals transmission levels as low as 30% (25×10^8 organisms) resulted in only 60% mortality.

From these experiments it would appear that in commercial mouse diets there is a substance (or substances) which increases the resistance of these animals to staphylococcal infections. Nearly all of the commercial diets contain a moderate proportion of materials derived from tissue sources. Since the antistaphylococcal agents discovered in

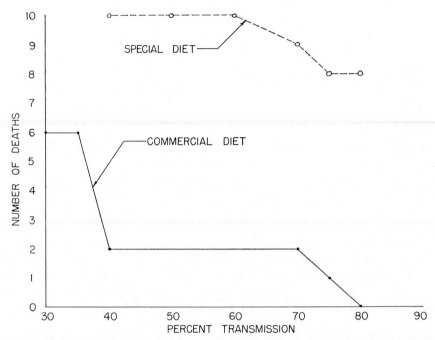

FIG. 7. EFFECT OF DIET ON THE SUSCEPTIBILITY OF BOONTUCKY MICE TO STAPHYLOCOCCAL INFECTION

our laboratories may be derived from animal tissues, it is possible that commercial diets contain them in small amounts. When commercial diet is ingested over a long period of time, the antistaphylococcic factor may be present in test animals in sufficient quantities to produce the enhanced resistance noted in the mice fed with one of the diets in our experiments.

Figure 8 represents the data obtained from the experiments conducted to evaluate the effect of genetic strain differences in mice on their degrees of susceptibility to S. aureus infections.

It is apparent from these results that the highly inbred strains of mice are the most susceptible to staphylococcal infections and that the susceptibility increases as the degree of inbreeding increases. It is also apparent that the inbred strains of mice showed a high degree of susceptibility even when fed a commercial diet. Their susceptibility therefore must be of such a level that the antistaphylococcic factors present in the commercial diet were not sufficient to overcome their weakness.

Table 32 is a summary chart of the experiments conducted with all strains of mice at all light transmission levels. It is of interest to note

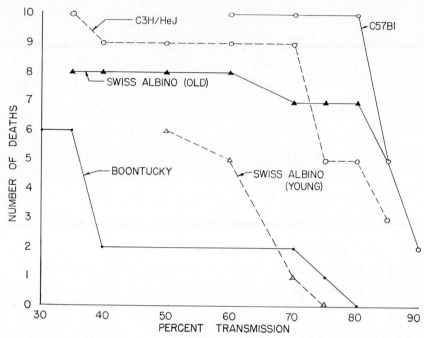

FIG. 8. SUSCEPTIBILITY OF FOUR STRAINS OF MICE TO *Staphylococcus aureus*
INFECTION

that with one strain of mice (the Swiss albino) age is also an apparent
determining factor of susceptibility, older mice succumbing to a much
lower dosage of organisms than younger ones. This is also clearly illustrated in Fig. 8. There is no apparent explanation for this occurrence
at the present time.

DISCUSSION

The foregoing data indicate that the susceptibility of a random-bred
strain of mice to staphylococcal infection can be considerably altered
by dietary changes. The data further indicate that susceptibility is also
dependent on the genetic strain of the mice and, that within the limits
of the experiments, the greater the degree of inbreeding, the greater the
susceptibility of the strain to infection.

A possible explanation for the former phenomenon may lie in the
fact that tissue materials incorporated in commercial mouse diets may
provide, in varying amounts, the probiotic factors which we have found
to be antistaphylococcal and capable of increasing the resistance of

TABLE 32

SUMMARY MORTALITY CHART FOR FOUR STRAINS OF MICE AT VARIOUS LIGHT TRANSMISSION
SUSPENSIONS OF ORGANISMS

Strain of Mice	Sex	Age (Weeks)	% Transmission	Mortality[3]	Expt.
c[1]-BT[2]	M	10–11	30	6/10	
c-BT	M	10–11	35	6/10	
C3H/HeJ	M	12–13	35	10/10	
Swiss	M	19–20	35	8/10	
c-BT	M	9–11	40	8/40	4
s[4]-BT	F	9–11	40	19/20	2
C3H/HeJ	M	10–13	40	18/20	2
Swiss	M	19–20	40	8/10	
s-BT	F	10–11	50	10/10	
Swiss	F	18–19	50	8/10	
Swiss	M	9–10	50	12/20	2
s-BT	F	10–11	60	20/20	2
C3H/HeJ	F, M	11–12, 16	60	28/30	3
Swiss	F, M	17, 18–19	60	24/30	3
Swiss	M	9–10	60	7/20	2
C57B1	M	7–8	60	10/10	
c-BT	M	9–11	70	6/30	3
s-BT	F	9–11	70	35/40	4
C3H/HeJ	F, M	11, 16–17	70	55/60	6
Swiss	F, M	18–19, 17	70	14/20	2
Swiss	M	9–10	70	1/20	2
C57B1	M	8–9	70	30/30	3
c-BT	M	9–10	75	1/10	
s-BT	M	9–10	75	8/10	
C3H/HeJ	M	12–14	75	5/10	
Swiss	M	14–15	75	7/10	
Swiss	M	9–10	75	0/10	
c-BT	M	9–10	80	0/10	
s-BT	M	9–10	80	8/10	
C3H/HeJ	M	12–14	80	5/10	
Swiss	F	14–15	80	7/10	
C57B1	F	7–8	80	10/10	
C3H/HeJ	M	12/13	85	3/10	
Swiss	F	14–15	85	5/10	
C57B1	F	7–8	85	5/10	
C57B1	F	7–8	90	2/10	

[1] Commercial diet.

[2] Boontucky strain of mice.

[3] First number indicates number of dead mice; second number, total number of mice in experiment.

[4] Special diet.

mice to this organism. In the corn, casein, methionine diet, used as a special diet in these experiments and in which tissue materials were omitted, the resistance of the mice was reduced, i.e., their susceptibility was increased.

The second observation—the relation of strain difference to suscepti-bility—might be explained on the basis that mice in general have, as an inherited characteristic, a high degree of susceptibility to *S. aureus* and that this weakness can be augmented by inbreeding. It is further evident that the inherited susceptibility of the inbred strains of mice, unlike the random bred, is of sufficient magnitude to withstand the inhibitory effect of the materials in commercial mouse diets.

Staphylococcal infections in mice have been attained with dosages of the organism sufficiently low to provide a suitable assay method which can be reasonably compared with staphylococcal studies in human beings. According to Elek (1956), staphylococcal doses of the order of 3×10^6 to 7×10^6 are required to produce pustular lesions in 100% of human subjects. By comparison, we have been able, by proper diet and strain selection, to produce mortalities in mice of 80 to 90% at organism dosages of 15×10^7 to 12×10^7.

REFERENCES

CHAPMAN, G. H. 1946. A single culture medium for selective isolation of plasma coagulating staphylococci and for improved testing for chromato- genesis, plasma coagulation, mannitol fermentation and the Stone reaction. J. Bacteriol. *51*, 409–410.

ELEK, S. D. 1956. Experimental staphylococcal infections in the skin of man. Ann. N. Y. Acad. Sci. *65*, 85–89.

HEALY, M. D. 1957. Biological and chemical studies on the hypoglycemic activity of *Eugenia jambolana*. Ph.D. Thesis, Institutum Divi Thomae.

CHAPTER 8

Identification of Active Principles

In previous chapters it has been demonstrated that probiotics can be isolated from a variety of tissues. However, the results of experiments up to this point would not indicate if probiotics from all tissues are the same; nor do the data show if there is one substance or if there are multiple substances which possess probiotic activity. Also, it is logical to inquire if it is the same substance that is effective against all susceptible organisms.

There is the further question of whether or not the probiotics which are effective therapeutically are the same as those which are effective prophylactically.

In order to answer some of these questions and to eliminate as many variables as possible, a series of researches was undertaken in which the crude extract from a single tissue, beef brain, was compared with several of its fractions and with pure, or related, compounds identified in the extract.

Using the crude brain extract, prepared as described in Chap. 1, as a starting material, a variety of fractionation procedures were investigated including the use of ion-exchange resins, column chromatography, thin layer chromatography, electrophoresis, and solvent extraction, or combinations of these. Only the more productive of these studies will be described.

In general the most useful procedures employed ion-exchange resins. These procedures indicated quite early that either an amphoteric substance, or both acid and basic substances, were associated with anti-staphylococcal activity. For example, we found that the active material was essentially stable between pH 2.5 and 9.0 and was also heat-stable. It was soluble in water and the more polar solvents. Passage of brain extract through the strong cation-exchange resin, Amberlite IR-100, followed by elution with dilute pyridine, increased the activity about tenfold, and 90% of the material was removed, including inorganic salts which constituted as much as 40% of some extracts. On the other hand, passage of the extract through the strong anion-exchanger, Amberlite IRA-400, followed by elution with $N/4$ hydrochloric acid also gave a potent preparation.

Paper chromatography revealed a number of amino acids. Identified at that time were aspartic acid, glutamic acid, glycine, alanine, arginine, histidine and γ-aminobutyric acid, as well as small peptides. Attempts to concentrate the activity of the pyridine eluate from Amberlite IR-100 on alumina were unsuccessful, and the use of cellulose columns gave little better success, although some concentration of activity was achieved and γ-aminobutyric acid was found to be the main constituent of the most active fraction. Use of the weak cation-exchanger, IRC-50, and dilute pyridine as the eluting agent also gave an active fraction which contained about 10% of γ-aminobutyric acid as the only ninhydrin-positive material. Tests at that time by the standard prophylactic assay procedure indicated that γ-aminobutyric acid was ineffective against experimental staphylococcal infections. Much later a "short-term" assay procedure showed that the amino acid did have activity but that its rapid metabolism or excretion probably prevented detection of activity by the older procedure in which there was a 24-hr period between the last administration of the drug and challenge with the organism. Consequently, it was concluded that ninhydrin-positive materials did not account for the antistaphylococcal activity.

For the time-being, a study was concentrated on acidic materials obtained by strongly acidifying crude brain extract with hydrochloric acid and repeatedly extracting with ether. This fraction (about 3.5% of the extract) was about 40 times as active as the parent extract. The acidified extract was then made strongly alkaline and extracted with ether. This basic fraction (about 1% of the extract) and the residue (about 9.5% of the extract) were both moderately active. The acid fraction was studied further and found to contain lactic and fumaric acids, both inactive against *S. aureus* infections. Reextracting of the acid fraction with ether at pH values of 7, 4.5, 2, and 1 in succession resulted in a ninetyfold increase in activity in the pH 4.5 fraction. The extracts obtained at pH 7 and pH 2 were slightly active, but the pH 1 extract was inactive and toxic. In addition to traces of lactic and fumaric acid the pH 4.5 fraction contained two unidentified acids. These were separated by developing a strip chromatogram with ethanol/concentrated ammonium hydroxide/water (80 : 5 : 15). Insufficient material was available for animal assay but the acid fractions were tested *in vitro* against *S. aureus* by the filter disc method and found to inhibit growth of the organism.

Because of the success of the Moore and Stein procedure for separating amino acids, attention was turned to the use of Dowex-50 W-X2 and elution with buffers of continuously increasing pH. These investigations showed that three fractions of brain extract, corresponding to the basic, neutral, and acidic amino acids, possessed marked antistaphylococcal activity, thus confirming the earlier indications of multiple active substances. We verified the existence of these active fractions by the use of electrophoresis, and undertook a detailed amino acid analysis by means of the automatic amino acid analyzer and microbiological procedures before and after hydrolysis of the brain extract; about 20 known amino acids and at least 10 other ninhydrin-positive substances were detected. One of the latter was identified as carnosine (β-alanylhistidine), a constituent of the basic fraction of brain extract.

Homocarnosine had previously been identified in brain by other workers (Pisano *et al.* 1961; Abraham *et al.* 1962; Kanazawa *et al.* 1965; Kanazawa and Sano 1967). By chromatography on an Amberlite CG-120 2,6-lutidine column followed by elution with 2,6-lutidine, diazotization, and measurement of absorption at 500 nm and by thin layer chromatography, we were able to identify and estimate carnosine and homocarnosine in brain extract.

Although many isolated experiments were performed on various pure compounds, the results of a group of experiments in which many of the compounds were compared simultaneously with crude brain extract are presented in order to simplify comparative evaluations. The compounds tested include homocarnosine sulfate, ϵ-aminocaproic acid, γ-aminobutyric acid, L-histidine hydrochloride (monohydrate), sphingomyelin, phrenosin, L-carnosine, L-anserine nitrate, δ-aminovaleric hydrochloride, L-1-methylhistidine (monohydrate) and 1-aminomethylcyclohexane-4-carboxylic acid.

MATERIALS AND METHODS

Experimental Animals

Throughout the course of these studies, Swiss albino mice, both male and female, were consistently used, except in a limited number of experiments for comparative purposes. The animals were between 10 and 14 weeks old and had an approximate average weight of 20–25 gm. These animals were raised and maintained mostly on the Rockland diet. Some experiments were conducted on animals raised on an experimental diet made in our own laboratories but were soon discontinued because of the lack of any significant advantage.

Organisms

Staphylococcus aureus.—Studies, both *in vivo* and *in vitro*, were conducted using penicillin-resistant strain, *S. aureus* Original, first isolated from a case of acute tonsilitis and maintained in our laboratories for a number of years. This strain is preserved in the lyophilized form and stored at 0° C. The lyophilized sample was first cultivated on sterile Difco SA 110 plates and then transferred to slants of the same medium. These slants after 24 hr of growth were stored under refrigeration (approximately 10° C) as the stock cultures. For all routine purposes, subcultures were made from the stock cultures on Difco SA 110. In our experience, one set of stock cultures could be maintained and used as long as 6 months beyond which growth was extremely poor on subculturing. However, there is no evidence that this drop in growth is associated with loss of virulence. Because of the loss of viability, the stock cultures were discarded and a fresh set was raised from the lyophilized sample. Virulence tests were done for each stock culture and only minor variations were noticed.

Inoculum.—Unless otherwise stated, the inoculum in all experiments was prepared from 24-hr cultures on sterile SA 110 slants at 37° C aerobically. The cells were washed and suspended in physiological saline (TC Tyrode Solution Difco) under aseptic conditions. Uniform dispersion was ensured by shaking vigorously with sterile glass beads in serum bottles. These suspensions were diluted further with adequate amounts of physiologic saline to give the desired light transmission when read on a nephelometer. From standard curves which had been established, the nephelometer readings could be converted to bacterial counts. The appropriate nephelometric reading (percent transmission) was predetermined for each stock culture initially by a process of trial and adjustments using different dilutions while ascertaining the virulence of the cultures. This was found to vary from 55 to 70% transmission.

A departure from conventional practice in bacteriology is the use of a dose of organisms that gives an LD_{80-90} instead of LD_{50} in these studies. This has been the practice in our laboratories in studies with staphylococci since lower dosages often fail to give consistent mortalities. After preparing the inoculum of the desired dilution to give an LD_{80-90}, 0.5 ml was inoculated subcutaneously in the groins of the animals.

Brain Extract: Prophylactic

A limited number of experiments were conducted to establish the prophylactic value against staphylococcal infections of a crude beef brain extract which was to be used as a standard for comparison. The experimental animals were given, subcutaneously, 20 mg of the brain extract per day for 5 days. On the sixth day they were challenged, along with a control group, with the predetermined LD_{80-90} mortality followed over a 5-day period. The results of one such experiment are recorded in Table 33.

In our present investigations variations in relative efficacy between different batches of brain extract have been noticed. Mortalities as high as 40% in experimental groups receiving 100 mg per animal, as compared to 90% in the controls, were obtained. However, in the majority of experiments, the mortality values showed a range of 0–30%. The efficiency of the crude brain extract may be affected by such factors as the age of the animals from which the brains were obtained, the relative freshness of the brain, etc.

Once the potency of the crude brain extract was established, attention was directed toward the assay of several different compounds for their possible prophylactic and therapeutic values.

TABLE 33

CRUDE BRAIN—PROPHYLACTIC—SUBCUTANEOUS

		Days Postchallenge				
		1	2	3	4	5
Group	Dose per Animal	% Mortality (10 Mice per Group)				
Control	—	50	60	90	90	90
Exptl.	100 mg	0	10	10	10	10

Screening Specific Compounds: Prophylactic

Aqueous solutions of the compounds in dosages indicated in Table 34 were administered subcutaneously to the respective experimental groups of animals in a three-day prophylactic series. Sphingomyelin and phrenosin are relatively insoluble in water, but were emulsified by warming gently and shaking vigorously. On the fourth day all the animals were challenged with the lethal dose of S. aureus. A control group was also used. The results of one such experiment are given in Table 34.

From several of the preliminary experiments with these compounds, it became apparent that homocarnosine was consistent in giving protection against subsequent challenge with S. aureus. Though not evident in the results recorded in Table 34, there were indications in other experiments that phrenosin was also worth considering in this respect. This was more encouraging in view of our recent findings that an active principle in the brain extract could be a cerebroside like phrenosin. In the light of the above screening tests, it was thought desirable to abandon some of the compounds assayed and concentrate on a few which included homocarnosine, L-carnosine, δ-aminovaleric acid, ε-aminocaproic acid,

TABLE 34

SPECIFIC COMPOUNDS—PROPHYLACTIC—SUBCUTANEOUS

Group	Dose per Animal in Mg	No. of Animals	Days Postchallenge				
			1	2	3	4	5
			% Mortality				
Control	—	10	50	50	60	60	60
Sphingomyelin	5	10	20	30	40	40	50
Phrenosin	5	10	20	40	40	50	50
Beta-Alanine	5	10	40	60	70	70	70
L-Histidine	10	10	50	70	90	90	90
L-1-Methylhistidine	5	9	44.4	55.5	66.6	66.6	66.6
Gamma-aminobutyric acid	5	10	80	90	100	100	100
Delta-aminovaleric acid	5	10	30	30	30	50	50
Epsilon-aminocaproic acid	5	9	44.4	55.5	55.5	55.5	66.6
L-Carnosine	10	10	40	60	60	60	70
Homocarnosine	5	10	20	30	30	30	30
Anserine	5	10	60	70	70	70	70
1-Aminomethylcyclohexane-4-carboxylic acid	5	10	60	60	60	80	80

phrenosin and sphingomyelin. The use of δ-aminovaleric acid and ε-aminocaproic acid was to see whether increasing molecular complexity is in any way related to the biological activity of the compounds under consideration. These compounds were administered in the same manner as before and the results after challenge are shown in Table 35.

These data further confirmed a definite value of homocarnosine in protecting Swiss albino mice against experimental staphylococcal infections. Consistent with the conclusions reached from earlier experiments, phrenosin, though less effective, also seems to possess some degree of protective activity.

An analysis of the results of several experiments revealed that experimental groups given L-carnosine, always exhibited mortalities higher than the control groups. Delta-aminovaleric acid and ε-aminocaproic acid

TABLE 35

SPECIFIC COMPOUND—PROPHYLACTIC—SUBCUTANEOUS

Group	Dose per Animal in Mg	Days Postchallenge				
		1	2	3	4	5
		% Mortality (10 Mice per Group)				
Control		50	70	80	80	90
Sphingomyelin	5	30	40	70	70	80
Phrenosin	5	10	30	40	40	40
δ-Amino-valeric acid	5	50	60	80	80	80
ε-Amino-caproic acid	5	40	70	70	70	70
L-Carnosine	10	70	100	100	100	100
Homocarnosine	5	20	30	30	30	30

were consistently ineffective. These therefore were abandoned from subsequent experiments, leaving only homocarnosine, phrenosin, and sphingomyelin to be considered for investigation.

However, a significant fact that became obvious at this point was that a high *in vivo* antistaphylococcal activity of sphingomyelin, which we had observed in C3H mice, could not be demonstrated in the Swiss albino mice. Therefore, it was decided to assay these compounds in different mouse strains to ascertain whether the discrepancies in results could be explained on the basis of host differences. Experiments were conducted on C3H female mice using sphingomyelin, phrenosin and homocarnosine in a three-day prophylactic series. Table 36 shows the results.

TABLE 36

SPHINGOMYELIN, PHRENOSIN AND HOMOCARNOSINE IN C3H MICE: PROPHYLACTIC

		Days Postchallenge				
	Dose per Animal in Mg	1	2	3	4	5
Group		% Mortality (10 Mice per Group)				
Control	—	10	70	100	100	100
Sphingomyelin	5	20	40	40	40	40
Phrenosin	5	70	70	70	70	70
Homocarnosine	5	20	40	40	40	40

Although the degree of protection by treatment with sphingomyelin in this experiment was less than those previously described, these studies do indicate that host differences may influence the *in vivo* activity of the compounds assayed. Homocarnosine, however, seems to be active in both strains of mice. Sphingomyelin and phrenosin seem to have a narrower host range of activity.

With the confirmation of the biological activities of homocarnosine and to some extent phrenosin, experiments were repeated in which these two compounds were compared with the crude brain extract. In addition, animals raised on the commercial and experimental diets were also compared. In all other respects the experiments are duplicates of the previous ones.

In this experiment (Table 37), sphingomyelin appears to be active in animals raised on the experimental diet. However, it must be emphasized that it is the only one in all our studies and was not confirmed in experiments before or after, on either diet in Swiss mice. This experiment also shows a variable behavior of phrenosin. However, the brain extract and homocarnosine are consistently active in both groups although there are some differences in the absolute degree of activity.

TABLE 37

BRAIN EXTRACT AND SPECIFIC COMPOUNDS COMPARED: PROPHYLACTIC

Group	Dose per Mouse in Mg	No. of Mice	Days Postchallenge				
			1	2	3	4	5
			% Mortality				
Experimental Diet							
Control	—	9	77.7	88.8	88.8	88.8	88.8
Brain extract	100	9	11.1	11.1	22.2	22.2	22.2
Sphingomyelin	5	7	14.2	14.2	14.2	14.2	14.2
Phrenosin	5	8	0	37.5	37.5	37.3	37.5
Homocarnosine	5	9	0	0	0	0	0
Commercial Diet							
Control	—	9	44.4	55.5	55.5	66.6	77.7
Brain extract	100	9	0	11.1	11.1	11.1	11.1
Sphingomyelin	5	7	42.6	71.0	71.0	71.0	71.0
Phrenosin	5	8	0	0	0	0	0
Homocarnosine	5	9	33.3	33.3	33.3	33.3	33.3

A comparative analysis of our data led us to the conclusion that in Swiss albino mice, homocarnosine is more effective in antistaphylococcal activity than phrenosin, when administered prophylactically, while spingomyelin is relatively ineffective. This is obvious in one typical experiment, the results of which are given in Table 38.

Homocarnosine and Phrenosin: Synergistic.—The consistent inactivity of sphingomyelin, led us to drop it from our remaining studies.

TABLE 38

HOMOCARNOSINE, PHRENOSIN AND SPHINGOMYELIN: PROPHYLACTIC

Group	Dose per Mouse in Mg	No. of Mice	Days Postchallenge				
			1	2	3	4	5
			% Mortality				
Control	—	10	40	50	50	60	60
Homocarnosine	5	9	0	0	0	0	11.1
Phrenosin	5	10	20	20	20	20	20
Sphingomyelin	5	9	33.3	44.4	44.4	44.4	44.4

One line of investigation at this point was to study the effect of homocarnosine and phrenosin together to ascertain whether there was any possible synergistic action *in vivo*. Experiments were conducted on animals on the experimental diet as well as those on the commercial diet. In each case, there were three experimental groups receiving homocarnosine, phrenosin, and a combination of homocarnosine and phrenosin in equal proportions. All were treated prophylactically for three days as before and the results, after challenge, are reported in Table 39.

TABLE 39

HOMOCARNOSINE AND PHRENOSIN—SYNERGISTIC—PROPHYLACTIC

Group	Dose per Mouse in Mg	Days Postchallenge				
		1	2	3	4	5
		% Mortality (9 Mice per Group)				
Experimental Diet						
Control	—	100	100	100	100	100
Homocarnosine	5	44.4	44.4	44.4	44.4	44.4
Phrenosin	5	55.5	55.5	66.6	66.6	66.6
Homocarnosine + Phrenosin	2.5 + 2.5	55.5	55.5	66.6	66.6	66.6
Commercial Diet						
Control	—	88.8	88.8	88.8	88.8	88.8
Homocarnosine	5	11.1	33.3	33.3	33.3	33.3
Phrenosin	5	22.2	33.3	44.4	44.4	44.4
Homocarnosine + Phrenosin	2.5 + 2.5	44.4	44.4	44.4	44.4	44.4

No synergistic action of homocarnosine and phrenosin was recognized although it may be mentioned that this type of study was not pursued in great detail. In Table 39, it will be seen that in both groups of mice, the mortalities in the groups which received a combination of homocarnosine and phrenosin was the same as in the group given phrenosin alone in the respective category. Although it is not possible to state categorically, from these limited experiments, that the combinations are no more effective than one of the compounds, it does seem safe to say that the effects are not additive.

By this time it became obvious that homocarnosine and brain extract compare very favorably in their prophylactic action in experimental staphylococcal infections in Swiss albino mice. Although mortality was taken as the criterion of reference, in all experiments these conclusions were corroborated by observations on other aspects of the infection, especially the nature and extent of the lesions produced, the time of healing and the general well-being of the animals. Although in some unusually good instances, homocarnosine prevented the development of lesions, in general the survivors of all groups did develop lesions of varying extent and severity. However, animals receiving brain extract and homocarnosine were marked by lesions of less severity and extent and also healed much faster (10–14 days) as compared to others.

The exploratory investigations, discussed thus far, led to a systematic elimination of most of the compounds with which the studies began. For reasons already mentioned, sphingomyelin, though reportedly active in some mouse strains, was dropped from our studies. Phrenosin, though effective, has shown a variable behavior. Homocarnosine, however, is consistently active. This consistent activity, the relative molecular simplicity as compared to phrenosin, and the availability in pure form, all set the stage for a much more intensive study of homocarnosine and the exclusion of all others, including phrenosin, from future experiments.

Of primary interest was to repeat the prophylactic experiments reported in the preceding pages, using the same dose of 5 mg per animal, given subcutaneously over 3 days. Since it is not necessary to reproduce the results of each individual experiment, a resumé of 25 experiments in which the mortalities ranged from 0 to 30% is represented in Table 40.

During the course of these studies, it became apparent that the homocarnosine available in the commercial form is not homogeneous in biological activity. This might, at least in part, account for the variations in mortalities in the various experiments. The best samples were

TABLE 40

HOMOCARNOSINE—PROPHYLACTIC—SUBCUTANEOUS (RESUMÉ)

Group	Dose per Mouse in Mg	No. Experiments	No. of Animals	% Mortality in 5 Days
Control	—	25	247	84.2
Exptl.	5	25	335	19.9

found to reduce mortalities as low as 0 to 10%. Some of the samples received from the suppliers were found to be even visibly heterogeneous; varying degrees of clumping and discoloration were observed. No attempt was made during these studies to check the chemical denaturation of the various commercial samples by chromatography or any other means.

In the following experiments each sample received was separately assayed before being used for comparative studies and in this way it was possible to obtain fairly consistent results.

Homocarnosine: Dose Determination.—Once the antistaphylococcal property of homocarnosine was established by an adequate number of experiments, it was important to determine the appropriate dose for optimum results. In all experiments reported above, an arbitrary dose of 5 mg per animal was used. However, no critical experiments were conducted to recommend this as the best dose. Three groups of animals were treated prophylactically in 3 days by the subcutaneous route as before with 5 mg, 2.5 mg, and 1.5 mg of homocarnosine per animal. The extent of protection given by the respective doses could be inferred from the mortality in five days recorded in Table 41.

These results suggest that, even with 1.5 mg per animal prophylactically, the protection against subsequent challenge is comparable with that of higher doses used before. This may be closer to the optimum than 5 mg or 2.5 mg. However, in view of the variations in results obtained with higher doses and the possibility of having a certain proportion of the sample in an inactive state (discussed before), it was thought desirable to continue to use a 5 mg dose in these investigations. Besides, there was absolutely no indication of any toxicity with homocarnosine at this dose, which further supported the use of this dose routinely.

Homocarnosine: Duration of Protection.—In experiments thus far, the animals were challenged within 24 hr after the termination of the prophylactic treatment and hence all the data refer only to the protection

TABLE 41

HOMOCARNOSINE—DOSE DETERMINATION—PROPHYLACTIC

			Days Postchallenge				
	Dose per		1	2	3	4	5
	Mouse	No. of					
Group	in Mg	Mice		% Mortality			
Control	—	10	70	80	80	80	90
Homocarnosine	5	20	0	5	5	5	5
Homocarnosine	2.5	20	10	10	10	10	10
Homocarnosine	1.5	10	10	20	20	20	20

within this narrow range of time. It was of interest to ascertain whether the protection given by the prophylactic administration of homocarnosine is only shortlived or longer lasting. A group of 50 mice were treated with homocarnosine (five milligrams per animal) in three subcutaneous injections. They were divided into five groups and each group was challenged with the lethal dose of S. aureus at weekly intervals, using a fresh set of controls each time. The first group was challenged 24 hr after the last treatment, as before. Mortalities in each group were recorded (Table 42) over periods of five days in each case.

Although there is a slight drop in protection with the lapse of time, there is enough evidence to indicate that homocarnosine by itself is able to protect mice against experimental staphylococcal infections at least up to a period of one month. It is clear from Table 42 that even in the last group challenged 28 days after treatment, the degree of protection is fairly comparable with results in many past experiments on immediate effects. In view of the fact that some degree of protection existed 28 days after treatment, experiments should be conducted covering longer periods of time.

Homocarnosine: Minimum Time for Expression.—As a corollary to the observations on the duration of protection, it was of interest to ascertain the minimum time after administration, required for homocarnosine to

TABLE 42

HOMOCARNOSINE—DURATION OF PROTECTION—PROPHYLACTIC

Group	No. of Animals	Days Postchallenge				
		1	2	3	4	5
		% Mortality				
Challenged 24 Hr After Treatment						
Control	10	70	70	70	80	80
Homocarnosine	10	0	0	0	10	10
Challenged 7 Days After Treatment						
Control	10	70	80	80	80	90
Homocarnosine	10	0	0	0	0	0
Challenged 14 Days After Treatment						
Control	10	70	90	90	90	90
Homocarnosine	10	20	20	20	20	20
Challenged 21 Days After Treatment						
Control	10	60	70	70	70	70
Homocarnosine	10	0	30	30	30	30
Challenged 28 Days After Treatment						
Control	9	66.6	77.7	77.7	77.7	77.7
Homocarnosine	9	22.2	22.2	22.2	22.2	22.2

express its activity. Fifty animals were treated with 5 mg of homocarnosine each, in one subcutaneous injection. They were divided into 5 groups of 10 each and successive groups were challenged at intervals of 1 hr, using a different control group each time. A fresh inoculum from a 24-hr culture was also used each time. Mortality in each group was recorded and compared against that of the control group (Table 43).

TABLE 43

HOMOCARNOSINE—MINIMUM TIME FOR EXPRESSION

Group	No. of Animals	Days Postchallenge				
		1	2	3	4	5
		% Mortality				
Challenged 1 Hr After Treatment						
Control	10	50	60	60	60	60
Homocarnosine	10	20	20	20	20	20
Challenged 2 Hr After Treatment						
Control	10	40	50	50	50	60
Homocarnosine	10	10	20	30	30	30
Challenged 3 Hr After Treatment						
Control	10	50	60	60	60	60
Homocarnosine	10	20	20	20	20	20
Challenged 4 Hr After Treatment						
Control	10	30	60	60	60	60
Homocarnosine	10	10	20	40	40	
Challenged 5 Hr After Treatment						
Control	10	50	50	50	50	50
Homocarnosine	10	10	10	10	10	10

Although the group challenged after 4 hr shows some inconsistency, there seems to be enough suggestive evidence that, even as early as 1 hr after treatment, homocarnosine is taken up by the animals and is able to express its antistaphylococcal property. In fact, the degree of protection compares well with that after 5 hr.

Is the Complete Peptide Necessary?—Earlier experiments indicate that though homocarnosine is effective in providing protection, its component, L-histidine, by itself is ineffective. Experiments were, therefore, designed to confirm this point and to see if the two together would have a synergistic effect or be antagonistic or merely be indifferent *in vivo*. It was thought that such an experiment might offer some clue to the molecular basis of the activity of homocarnosine.

Since molar concentrations offer a better standard for comparison, these substances were administered in equimolar proportions. Three

TABLE 44

HOMOCARNOSINE + L-HISTIDINE: PROPHYLACTIC

			Days Postchallenge				
			1	2	3	4	5
Group	Dose per Mouse in μM	No. of Mice	% Mortality (10 Mice per Group)				
Control	—		80	80	80	80	80
L-Histidine	15		80	80	80	80	80
Homocarnosine	15		0	10	10	10	10
L-Histidine + Homocarnosine	15 + 15		30	50	50	60	60

experimental groups of animals were treated prophylactically in three days, each group receiving per animal: (1) 15 μM L-histidine; (2) 15 μM homocarnosine; and (3) 15 μM L-histidine + 15 μM homocarnosine. This dosage was used since 5 mg of homocarnosine routinely used in our previous experiments is approximately equivalent to 15 μM. Mortality in the various groups was recorded daily for five days (Table 44).

A significant point worth mentioning is the fact that L-histidine when administered with homocarnosine, nearly offsets the antistaphylococcal property of the latter. Since homocarnosine is a dipeptide of L-histidine and γ-aminobutyric acid, a more extended experiment was then performed to compare the activity of homocarnosine with both the components as well as to ascertain the action of the two components themselves when administered in equimolar ratios. Experimental groups also were included to study the effect of homocarnosine in combination with either of the constituents. The results of this experiment are recorded in Table 45.

TABLE 45
HOMOCARNOSINE, L-HISTIDINE AND GAMMA-AMINOBUTYRIC ACID: PROPHYLACTIC

Group	Dose per Mouse in μM	No. of Mice	Days Postchallenge 1	2	3	4	6
			% Mortality				
Control	—	10	90	90	90	90	90
L-Histidine	15	10	80	80	80	80	80
Gamma-amino-butyric acid	15	10	40	70	70	80	80
L-Histidine + gamma-aminobutyric acid	15 + 15	10	70	70	80	80	80
Homocarnosine	15	10	20	20	20	20	20
Homocarnosine + L-histidine	15 + 15	10	10	50	60	60	60
Homocarnosine + gamma-amino-butyric acid	15 + 15	10	50	60	70	70	70

These experiments clearly indicate that while homocarnosine is effective in providing protection against the infection, the components L-histidine and γ-aminobutyric acid either singly or in combination (administered in the same ratios as in the whole peptide) are ineffective. Obviously, under the conditions of our experiment, the animals are not able to conjugate the components into homocarnosine. However, far more significant is the finding that either of the components, L-histidine or γ-aminobutyric acid, offsets or interferes with, the biological activity of the complete peptide. This interference seems to express itself much faster in the case of γ-aminobutyric acid, while L-histidine does the same in a rather delayed manner as borne out by these experiments.

Homocarnosine: Therapeutic.—A few experiments were conducted to ascertain if homocarnosine displays any therapeutic value. Two groups of animals—one control, the other experimental—were challenged with the predetermined lethal dose of *S. aureus.* The experimental animals were given a subcutaneous injection of 0.33 ml of an aqueous solution of homocarnosine (5 mg/ml) simultaneously with the challenge. The same dose of homocarnosine was repeated after every 6 hr. Mortality was recorded for a period of five days (Table 46).

In this experiment, the animals received only 3 doses of homocarnosine equivalent to 5 mg per animal. Although the mortality in the first 24-hr period was low as compared to the control group, the animals looked very sick, their physical condition not permitting any further treatment. Even those animals which survived beyond the five-day period of the experiment did not show any signs of recovery.

TABLE 46

HOMOCARNOSINE: THERAPEUTIC

Group	No. of Animals	Days Postchallenge				
		1	2	3	4	5
		% Mortality				
Control	10	80	80	90	90	90
Exptl.	10	30	50	50	50	50

Since the crude brain extract has been shown to be effective both prophylactically and therapeutically, from these results it seems hardly probable that homocarnosine and the other pure compounds tested are the sole source of activity of brain extract.

SALMONELLA TYPHI

Having observed that crude brain extract which is effective against *S. aureus* is also effective against *Salmonella typhi*, experiments were undertaken in which the activity of fractions of crude brain extract and some pure compounds were compared with crude brain extract in effectiveness against artificially induced *Salmonella* infections in mice. Such experiments were based on a prophylactic plan of inoculation.

Swiss albino male and female mice, ranging in age between 13 and 21 weeks, were used. Each experiment consisted of three groups of 10 mice per group. Animals treated with homocarnosine sulfate received 5 mg subcutaneously daily for five consecutive days, or a total of 25 mg. Animals treated with crude brain extract received 20 mg subcutaneously daily for 5 days, or a total of 100 mg. On the fifth day, 2 to 3 hr after the last injection, the experimental groups and a control group received an LD_{50} challenge dose of *Salmonella* obtained from a 24-hr culture. Table 47 gives the results of these experiments.

TABLE 47

SERIES ASSAY OF HOMOCARNOSINE VS CRUDE BRAIN EXTRACT AGAINST *Salmonella typhi* INFECTIONS IN SWISS ALBINO MICE

Sex	% Mortality (10 Mice per Group)		
	Homo[1]	Cr Brain[2]	Control
Female	20	10	60
Female	20	20	70
Female	10	10	40
Male	10	10	40

[1] Homo = Homocarnosine.
[2] Cr Brain = Crude Brain.

At the dosages used, the activity of homocarnosine is, in some instances, equal to that of the crude brain extract against *Salmonella* infection in mice.

The acidic portion of crude brain material can be further divided into fractions according to the degree of acidity. The preparation of three such acidic fractions led to the identification of a variety of compounds including glutathione (oxidized), glutathione (reduced), cysteic acid, taurine, and phosphoethanolamine. Only two of these pure compounds were tested for their effect on artificially induced infection, namely, glutathione (oxidized) and phosphoethanolamine. Glutathione (oxidized) was chosen since it exhibited a chemical relationship to all the other compounds isolated with the exception of phosphoethanolamine and the latter was chosen for its lack of relationship.

As in previous experiments, Swiss albino males and females, raised on the semipurified synthetic diet, were used. The dosage of the compounds was determined by their relative percentage in 1 ml of brain tissue. On this basis the dosage of glutathione (oxidized) was set at 0.1 mg/mouse/day for 5 days, or a total of 0.5 mg. The dosage of phosphoethanolamine was 0.2 mg/mouse/day for 5 days, or a total of 1.0 mg. On the fifth day, 2 to 3 hr after the last injection, the experimental groups and a control group received an LD_{50} challenge dose of *Salmonella* obtained from a 24-hr culture. The results of this study are shown in Table 48.

From the results presented, it is evident that no beneficial effect is obtained with glutathione or phosphoethanolamine in prophylactic treatment against *Salmonella* infection in mice.

TABLE 48

COMPARISON OF GLUTATHIONE AND PHOSPHOETHANOLAMINE WITH CRUDE BRAIN EXTRACT AGAINST *Salmonella typhi* INFECTION IN SWISS ALBINO MICE

Sex	Material	% Mortality (10 Mice per Group)		
		Exptl.	Crude Brain	Control
Female	Gluta[1]	70	20	70
Female	Gluta	50	10	60
Male	Gluta	50	10	40
Female	Gluta	100	30	50
Female	PEA[2]	60	10	60
Female	PEA	90	10	60
Male	PEA	50	10	40
Female	PEA	80	30	50

[1] Gluta = Glutathione.
[2] PEA = Phosphoethanolamine.

VIRUSES

Having established a significant degree of protection of mice to induced encephalomyocarditis infections, by the subcutaneous injection of crude brain extract, investigations were extended to include a study of fractions of the active materials. Several pure compounds, which previously had been shown to be present in the crude brain extract, some of which we had shown to be effective against certain bacterial infections, were tested against viral infections. The materials used included homocarnosine, glutathione (oxidized), phosphoethanolamine and hydrolyzed brain extract fraction.

The hydrolyzed fraction was prepared in the following manner: Equal portions of crude brain extract and 36.5% hydrochloric acid were placed in a pyrex tube and sealed by fusing. This tube was placed in an oven at 105°–110° C for 24 hr. The product of this hydrolysis was passed through a ground glass filter. The filtrate was evaporated to dryness under reduced pressure and reconstituted with distilled water. The process was repeated several times to ensure the exclusion of hydrochloric acid. The final reconstituted product was concentrated by glass distillation, the pH adjusted to 7, the salts removed by passage through a Sephadex G-10 column, passed through a Seitz filter, its dry weight determined, and then bottled for testing.

Homocarnosine was tested for possible activity against artificially induced EMC virus infection in mice. A series of prophylactic experiments was conducted in which treatment inoculations were given subcutaneously for five successive days. Each animal received 5 mg of homocarnosine per injection, or a total of 25 mg. A group of animals, receiving the same treatment with crude brain extract at a dosage of 20 mg per mouse per injection, was introduced for the purpose of comparing its activity with that of homocarnosine. Boontucky male and female mice, ranging in age from 3 to 4 weeks, were used in this assay series. The results of these investigations, recorded in Table 49, illustrate the degree of protection afforded by homocarnosine.

Glutathione (oxidized), phosphoethanolamine, and the hydrolyzed fraction were assayed together since all three are contained in the acidic portion of crude brain extract. These materials were tested prophylactically, using BT male and female mice ranging from 3 to 4 weeks old. The dosage level (per injection) for glutathione (oxidized) and phosphoethanolamine was 0.1 mg and 0.2 mg respectively. These dosages were determined by the relative percentage of these compounds in 1 ml of brain tissue. Since the hydrolyzed fraction was assayed to

TABLE 49

COMPARISON OF HOMOCARNOSINE AND CRUDE BRAIN EXTRACT
AGAINST EMC VIRUS INFECTION IN BT MICE

	% Mortality (10 Mice per Group)		
Sex	Homo[1]	Control	Cr Brain[2]
Female	10	60	10
Male	50	70	40
Female	40	40	0
Male	20	40	—

[1] Homo = Homocarnosine.
[2] Cr Brain = Crude Brain.

determine whether any activity existed after such treatment of crude brain material, the dosage level was set at 20 mg per injection, the same as crude brain extract. After 5 treatments with the test material, all animals, including the control group, were inoculated intraperitoneally with 0.25 ml of a $10^{-8.2}$ dilution of EMC virus. The results of this series of assays are recorded in Table 50.

It will be noted that the three pure compounds, including the hydrolyzed test fraction, demonstrate a certain degree of activity. Although the activity of these substances does not surpass that of the crude brain extract, the existence of a possible relationship must be considered.

Prophylactic administration of homocarnosine injected subcutaneously resulted in significant protection of mice against EMC viral infection. A similar effect was noted in animals treated prophylactically with glutathione (oxidized). Treatment with glutathione (oxidized) gave

TABLE 50

COMPARISON OF GLUTATHIONE (OXIDIZED), PHOSPHOETHANOLAMINE, HYDRO-
LYZED FRACTION OF CRUDE BRAIN EXTRACT AND CRUDE BRAIN EXTRACT
AGAINST EMC VIRUS INFECTION IN BT MICE

		% Mortality (19 Mice per Group)		
Sex	Test Material	Exptl.	Control	Cr Brain[1]
Male	GSSG[2]	20	60	10
Female	GSSG	30	70	40
Female	GSSG	40	40	0
Male	GSSG	10	40	—
Male	PEA[3]	30	60	10
Female	PEA	20	40	0
Female	PEA	50	70	40
Male	PEA	0	40	—
Female	HYDTF[4]	0	40	0
Male	HYDTF	20	50	10

[1] Cr Brain = Crude Brain.
[2] GSSG = Glutathione (oxidized).
[3] PEA = Phosphoethanolamine.
[4] HYDTF = Hydrolyzed Test Fraction.

an average protection of 57%. Likewise, phosphoethanolamine gave an average protection of 57%.

The hydrolyzed fraction was included primarily to determine if any activity remained in the crude brain extract after treatment. In the experiments in which it was used, it afforded protection of 100% and 60% compared to 100% and 80% by the nonhydrolyzed crude brain extract.

Although the three pure compounds and the hydrolyzed test fraction demonstrated a certain degree of activity, none equaled that of the crude brain extract. This fact may be an indication that the effect of crude brain extract is not due to any one pure component, but may be a complex interaction of several of these components, or possibly other compounds not yet tested.

The fact that activity is retained after hydrolysis, as demonstrated by the protection percentages of the hydrolyzed fraction, seems to indicate that a major portion of the activity may reside in the simple amino acids of the brain extract. However, a certain amount of activity in the whole brain extract may also be attributed to small peptides because a certain degree of protection was also obtained by treatment of infected animals with homocarnosine.

REFERENCES

ABRAHAM, D., PISANO, J. J., and UDENFRIEND, S. 1962. The distribution of homocarnosine in mammals. Arch. Biochem. Biophys. 99, 210–213.

KANAZAWA, A., KAKIMOTO, Y., MIYAMOTO, E., and SANO, I. 1965. Isolation and identification of homocarnosine from bovine brain. J. Neurochem. 12, 957–958.

KANAZAWA, A., and SANO, I. 1967. A method of determination of homocarnosine and its distribution in mammalian tissues. J. Neurochem. 14, 211–214.

PISANO, J. J. et al. 1961. Isolation of γ-aminobutyrylhistidine (homocarnosine) from brain. J. Biol. Chem. 236, 499–502.

CHAPTER 9

Search for Host Reactions to Probiotics

It has been shown that it is the protein-free fraction isolated from organs, and synthetic nonprotein compounds which are effective prophylactically and therapeutically in protecting the host against certain bacterial and viral diseases.

It will be recalled that some of the effective crude extracts, when tested *in vitro*, are toxic for some bacteria, and nontoxic for others. For the present only those substances will be considered which are nontoxic when tested *in vitro* against the pathogen to be studied, but prophylactically or therapeutically effective against it.

Having discovered little of value to shed light on the mechanism of action of probiotics from studies of the action of these substances on microorganisms, the possible effect of probiotics on the host will be considered.

Since probiotics are prepared as protein-free extracts, and since nonprotein compounds such as homocarnosine, are therapeutically effective, the possibility that they may act through the mechanism of antibody formation seems remote. However, since our understanding of the method by which antibodies produce their effects is by no means complete, there would be no justification for ignoring the possibility of a relationship existing between probiotics and antibodies.

The well-established fact that the symptoms of a disease may disappear well before the antibody level has reached a maximum lends support to the theory that even in immunity which results from a reaction to a foreign protein there are other factors which play a part in controlling the disease.

Experiments reported by Kahn (1934) indicate that tissue reactions to foreign proteins may occur in the absence of antibodies. He was able to demonstrate that different tissues of nonimmune rabbits possessed different localizing capacities for tissue-injected foreign proteins. Also, on the injection of a foreign protein in nonimmune rabbits, the localizing response of the skin to the specific protein increased from day to day during the incubation period, whereas precipitins first appeared at the end of the incubation period. Furthermore, these precipitins generally disappeared from the blood stream in about one week, while the localizing response remained for several weeks (Kahn, 1936).

Kahn *et al.* (1956) have observed that Arthus reactions in different areas of the rabbit's skin markedly differ in intensity. The reactions are very severe in the back and in the facial area, mild in the abdominal area and practically negative in the groin. The fact that probiotics are effective therapeutically as well as prophylactically must be taken into consideration.

In a search for a possible explanation of the prophylactic properties of probiotics, comparative tests for the accepted immune reactions were conducted on animals before and after resistance was induced by the use of probiotics. Since, in no instance in repeated experiments was there any indication of a correlation of the actions of probiotics and known immunological reactions, the detailed data would have little significance and hence have been omitted from this presentation.

RESISTANCE TO RECHALLENGE

Another search for information which it was felt might lead to an understanding of the action of probiotics was through a study of the duration of resistance to rechallenge of animals previously rendered immune by probiotic treatment.

Data have already been presented which show that administration of homocarnosine alone induces resistance to staphylococcal infections in mice at least up to a period of one month. In view of the relatively frequent recurrence of staphylococcal infections, as stated previously, if immunity to this organism develops as a result of infection, it must be short-lived or only partial.

It was therefore of interest to compare survivors from groups treated with crude brain extract, homocarnosine, sphingomyelin and phrenosin for resistance to rechallenge to the same organism.

The survivors after the first challenge in the respective groups were maintained under identical conditions, and after appropriate intervals they were rechallenged with the lethal dose of *Staphylococcus aureus*. Fresh control groups were employed in each test. Mortality in each group was taken as an index of relative resistance or susceptibility. Essentially the same results were obtained in repeated experiments and the results of one such experiment are reproduced in Table 51. In this particular case the animals were raised on the semipurified synthetic diet and were rechallenged 59 days after the first challenge.

Table 52 represents the results of a similar experiment with the exception that the animals were those on the commercial diet and that the comparisons are restricted to homocarnosine and phrenosin sepa-

TABLE 51

SURVIVORS RECHALLENGED 59 DAYS AFTER THE FIRST CHALLENGE

Group	No. of Animals	Mortality in Days Postchallenge, %				
		1	2	3	4	5
Control	10	100	100	100	100	100
Survivors from brain extract	7	14.2	14.2	14.2	14.2	14.2
Survivors from sphingomyelin	5	0	0	0	0	0
Survivors from phrenosin	4	0	0	0	0	0
Survivors from homocarnosine	8	0	0	0	0	0

rately as well as in combination. Animals which survived the first challenge following treatment with phrenosin, homocarnosine, and a combination of the two were rechallenged 41 days after the first challenge using a control group for comparison.

These rechallenge experiments were performed at varying intervals after the first challenge up to a maximum of 59 days and it was observed that consistently, irrespective of the treatment prior to challenge, the survivors showed almost complete immunity at least up to the periods covered in our experiments. It may be mentioned that in some experiments an occasional animal died but such deaths were extremely rare as to be of negligible importance. However, these do not tell whether the immunity observed is the result of the first challenge or is directly related to the biological activity of the compounds used. It was felt

TABLE 52

SURVIVORS RECHALLENGED 41 DAYS AFTER THE FIRST CHALLENGE

Group	No. of Animals	Mortality in Days Postchallenge, %				
		1	2	3	4	5
Control	10	80	90	90	90	90
Survivors from phrenosin	5	0	0	0	0	0
Survivors from homocarnosine	5	0	0	0	0	0
Survivors from phrenosin + homocarnosine	5	0	0	0	0	0

at this point that the observed resistance is perhaps the result of the first infection or of a preexisting resistance such as demonstrated itself in the surviving controls. This could be satisfactorily explained only by rechallenging survivors from untreated controls. Accordingly, such experiments were performed and typical results are recorded in Table 53. In this particular experiment the animals were rechallenged 26 days after the first challenge.

The results of several of these experiments were comparable and demonstrated complete immunity to reinfection at different intervals

TABLE 53
ACQUIRED RESISTANCE AFTER ACTIVE INFECTION

Group	No. of Animals	Mortality in Days Postchallenge, %				
		1	2	3	4	5
Control	10	90	90	90	90	90
Survivors from infection	10	0	0	0	0	0

after the first challenge. However, the maximum limit of this acquired immunity following active infection was not ascertained. At any rate, there is enough evidence to suggest that preattained resistance, or infection by itself could account for some of the immunity to rechallenge.

"Immune" Serum *in Vitro*

Serum from animals that survived an infection after treatment with homocarnosine, was used in experiments *in vitro,* for possible effects on the organisms. In preliminary experiments, the effects of "immune" serum and normal serum (serum from untreated, uninfected animals) on the capacity to ferment mannitol and liquefy gelatin as well as to produce pigment and coagulase were studied. In all instances 0.5 ml of the sterile serum was incorporated into 5 ml of the respective test media and appropriate controls were used in each case. All the tests were performed by the methods previously described. Table 54 is a resume of these studies and illustrates the inability of "immune" serum to alter the characteristics examined.

TABLE 54
"IMMUNE" SERUM: EFFECT OF BIOCHEMICAL CHARACTERISTICS

Material Tested	Coagulase Production	Mannitol Fermentation	Pigment Production	Gelatin Liquefaction
None (Control)	+	+	+	+
Normal serum	+	+	+	+
"Immune" serum	+	+	+	+

It was then decided to investigate the possibility of a bactericidal effect of the "immune" serum. Initial studies were carried out by soaking sterile filter paper discs in plates seeded with the organisms and incubating for periods up to 72 hr. These discs, which were 0.5 cm in diameter, were soaked with 0.1 ml of the test serum. In the control sets, the discs were soaked with the same amount of physiological saline. It was observed that the growth around both of the discs soaked in the normal and "immune" sera was considerably more dense than that around the control discs, and was even overgrown by the organisms.

These observations suggested that both normal and "immune" sera are similar at least in that they are growth promoters *in vitro*.

More precise growth studies were then undertaken using the basal medium (liquid) containing 12 supplementing amino acids. Tubes were set up with 7.5 ml of the medium to which were added 0.5 ml of the "immune" serum. Control tubes were used in which the serum was replaced by saline. All were inoculated with 2 drops of a saline suspension of twice-washed cells of *S. aureus* adjusted to 95% light transmission. Using the turbidimetric readings at successive intervals, growth curves were constructed (Fig. 9).

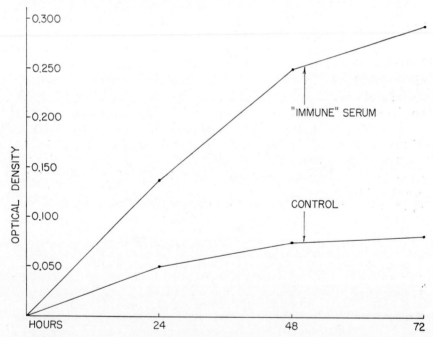

FIG. 9. EFFECT OF "IMMUNE" SERUM ON GROWTH OF *Staphylococcus aureus In Vitro*

There is a very marked and definite stimulation of growth by the "immune" serum. Similar stimulatory results were obtained for the normal serum as well. Figure 10 represents the results of an experiment performed in the same way and illustrates the stimulation of growth by normal and "immune" sera. These results clearly suggest that "immune" serum does not have any bactericidal or bacteriostatic properties but acts as a growth promotor *in vitro* and resembles the normal serum.

Transfer of "Immune" Serum.—Immunity to rechallenge suggested the need for another study of the "immune" animal itself. The most obvious choice was to examine the sera of these animals. "Immune" serum in this discussion is used in a restricted sense and refers to the serum of those animals resistant to rechallenge.

Blood from several resistant animals was drawn by the orbital bleeding technique using capillary hematocrit tubes. Each animal was bled to death and all blood was pooled in centrifuge tubes and allowed to clot by standing at room temperature for approximately 30 min. The clot was then loosened with a spatula and centrifuged for 12 min at

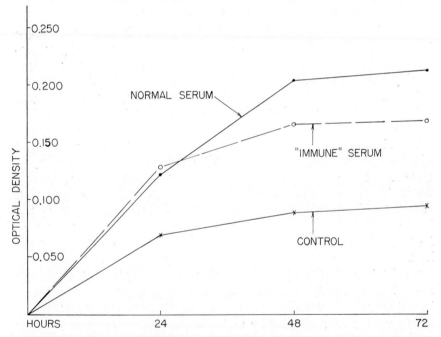

Fig. 10. COMPARATIVE EFFECTS OF "IMMUNE" AND NORMAL SERA ON GROWTH OF *Staphylococcus aureus In Vitro*

1700 rpm in an ordinary clinical centrifuge. The clear supernatant serum was drawn off carefully by a sterile Pasteur pipette.

In some instances a second centrifugation was employed to ensure the removal of all cells and debris. The serum was sterilized by passing through sterile Millipore filters and stored in sterile serum bottles at 10° C. As far as possible, fresh serum was used in all experiments. The maximum period of storage was 10 days beyond which the unused samples were discarded.

Experiments were conducted to ascertain whether the passive transfer of immunity is possible. The experimental animals were given 0.2 ml each of "immune" serum intravenously (through the tail vein) and the control group was given an equivalent volume of physiological saline. They were challenged 24 hr later with the lethal dose of S. *aureus* and the mortalities were recorded.

The results of the several tests are not presented here since the difference between experimental and control animals was not significant and it was concluded that the immunity resulting from the use of probiotics is not transferable passively.

EFFECT OF PROBIOTICS ON PROPERDIN LEVEL

It has been recognized that there exists a type of protection against infection, or a type of resistance which transcends the limits of antigenic specificity, and from time to time this kind of resistance to infection has been observed, even though demonstrable antibodies could not be detected. Though the level of resistance achieved in this way was at times small, it was sufficient to indicate that it might nonetheless contribute to immunity.

The observations mentioned began with some early work in the field of microbiology and were first noted by Kolle and Prigge (1929). In more recent literature, which has been summarized by Brandis (1954), the rapid production of a protective effect against challenge with *Salmonella derby* by the injection into mice of unrelated products has been reported. He called his effect "proimmunity" and considered it to be the result of nonspecific stimulation of the cellular defenses of the host.

Landsteiner (1945) stated that substances not identical with, but somewhat analogous to, specifically acquired antibodies, are produced in certain animals without any relationship to antigenic stimuli. These substances are characterized by their low order specificity and by their weak union with antigens.

The role of complement $C'1$, $C'2$, $C'3$ and $C'4$ in natural immunity reactions has also received a great deal of attention (Kolle and Prigge 1929; Pillemer 1943; Osborne 1937; and Zinsser *et al.* 1946). In an attempt to isolate one of the four components, namely $C'3$, a new serum protein, properdin (Pillemer *et al.* 1954A), an important factor in natural immunity, was discovered and isolated.

Certain bacteria and bacterial products, as well as other substances such as lipopolysaccharides, were shown to interact with the properdin system *in vitro* and to alter properdin levels *in vivo* (Pillemer *et al.*

1955). Further studies on properdin (Pillemer *et al.* 1954B) showed it to be a euglobulin with a molecular weight at least 8 times that of gamma globulin, and representing not more than 0.03% of the total serum protein. Normal human and other mammalian sera were shown to contain properdin (Pillemer 1955; Pillemer *et al.* 1954A), an important constituent of the natural defense of the blood. Properdin, in conjunction with complement and magnesium ions, participates in the destruction of certain bacteria, the inactivation of viruses, and the destruction of abnormal erythrocytes.

Thus, it has been pointed out that properdin differs from antibodies in many respects, and in particular in its apparent lack of serological specificity, its requirements for magnesium ions and complement for its interactions, and its physical and chemical properties. It has been generally concluded that alterations in the serum properdin levels *in vivo* appear to influence the course of certain experimental infections (Rowley, 1955).

In view of the protective effect of deproteinized beef tissue extracts on induced staphylococcal infections in mice, and the researches which indicated that this protective effect was independent of any increase in the normal specific immune defense mechanisms, the decision was made to determine whether or not the properdin levels in experimental animals, treated with beef tissue extracts and which were subsequently observed to be resistant to challenge doses of *S. aureus*, were affected. It was hoped that this work might add to our knowledge of the mechanism of action of probiotics in controlling infections.

The study that follows is therefore concerned with a more complete characterization of the increased resistance to staphylococcal infections that has been observed in mice following treatment with beef tissue extract preparations.

Particular attention is directed toward the dose, the timing of its administration, and the duration of the ensuing resistance. Definite information is presented on the relationship of properdin titers after treatment to the ability of the host to resist infections that have been induced with a strain of *S. aureus* in experimental animals.

Determination of the Serum Properdin Levels in Mice Prior to, and at Varying Intervals After Treatment with Deproteinized Beef Spleen Extract

In order to determine whether probiotics would have any effect on the serum properdin levels in the experimental animal, several groups of normal Boontucky white mice ranging in age from 9–12 weeks, consisting of a mixture of male and female animals in each group, were inoculated subcutaneously with 100 mg of beef spleen extract which was designated SSBK-2. Thereafter, each group consisting of ten animals was exsanguinated at definite intervals, and their blood pooled to form a single serum specimen for the properdin titration.

TABLE 55

RESULTS OF THE SERUM PROPERDIN LEVELS IN MICE PRIOR TO, AND AFTER TREATMENT WITH SUPERNATE BEEF SPLEEN TISSUE EXTRACT SSBK-2

No. of Animals	Hours After Treatment	Units of Properdin per Ml of Serum
10	0	12
10	3	15
10	6	14
10	12	14
10	18	15
10	24	12
10	36	12
10	48	12

Table 55 shows the properdin levels as determined over the experimental period of 48 hr. The differences in titers of the various groups after treatment were within the limits of the normal range as established previously when the test was carried out on animals which had received no form of prior treatment. Thus, the effect of the tissue extract SSBK-2 on the properdin levels in the experimental animals was considered negligible.

Comparison of Mortality and Serum Properdin Levels in Untreated and Treated Animals After Challenge with *Staphylococcus aureus*

In order to investigate further the possible relationship of properdin to the resistance induced by probiotics, a series of experiments was conducted in which the mortality and serum properdin levels of treated and untreated animals were compared after intraperitoneal challenge with the standardized lethal suspension of *S. aureus*.

Twelve groups of white mice ranging in age from 8–10 weeks and consisting of both male and female animals were subdivided into 2 sets of 6 groups, one set serving as the experimental groups and the other as the control groups. Each individual group in both sets consisted of from 10 to 30 animals. All animals belonging to the experimental groups were subcutaneously inoculated with 100 mg of the splenic tissue extract SSBK-2, and challenged intraperitoneally 24 hr after treatment with 0.5 ml of a standardized lethal suspension of *S. aureus*. Each of the

TABLE 56

THE PERCENT MORTALITY AND SERUM PROPERDIN LEVELS IN UNTREATED AND
SUBCUTANEOUSLY TREATED ANIMALS AFTER INTRAPERITONEAL CHALLENGE
WITH A STANDARDIZED SUSPENSION OF *Staphylococcus aureus*

Number of Animals	Hours Post-challenge	% Mortality		Units Properdin/Ml	
		Untreated	Treated	Untreated	Treated
10	0	0	0	14	12
10	3	0	0	10	14
10	6	10	0	12	9
20	12	40	30	5	5
30	18	70	40	3	8
30	24	80	40	3	12

remaining six groups of animals which served as the untreated controls
was challenged at the same time with an identical volume of the culture
suspension. At varying intervals after challenge, the survivors from one
group each of the treated and untreated animals were exsanguinated,
their blood pooled to form individual experimental and control group
serum specimens for properdin determinations and the mortalities in
each group recorded. Two separate experiments were conducted.

The results of these determinations over a period of 24 hr, are shown
in Tables 56 and 57, and Fig. 11 and 12. The data afford a suitable comparison of the effect of treatment plus challenge on the one hand, and
challenge without treatment on the other. There are indications of a
gradual fall in properdin titer during the first 12 hr after challenge in
both the treated and untreated groups. Thereafter a gradual rise in titer
12–24 hr after challenge in the treated groups appears to differentiate
them from the the untreated groups where a fall in titer appears to take
place during the same period. This rise in properdin titer in the treated
groups appeared to be associated with an increase in resistance when
compared to the progressive fall in titer within the untreated groups
which were more susceptible to the experimentally induced *Staphylo-*

TABLE 57

THE PERCENT MORTALITY AND SERUM PROPERDIN LEVELS IN UNTREATED AND
SUBCUTANEOUSLY TREATED ANIMALS AFTER INTRAPERITONEAL CHALLENGE
WITH A STANDARDIZED SUSPENSION OF *Staphylococcus aureus*

Number of Animals	Hours Post-challenge	% Mortality		Units Properdin/Ml	
		Untreated	Treated	Untreated	Treated
10	0	0	0	14	14
10	3	0	0	14	12
10	6	10	10	12	12
20	12	50	10	6	8
30	18	80	40	4	9
30	24	90	50	2	12

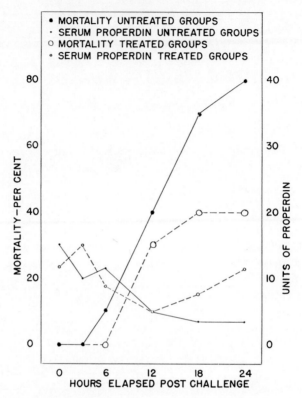

FIG. 11. PERCENT MORTALITY AND SERUM PROPERDIN LEVELS IN UNTREATED AND SUBCUTANEOUSLY TREATED ANIMALS AFTER INTRAPERITONEAL CHALLENGE WITH A STANDARDIZED SUSPENSION OF *Staphylococcus aureus*. EXPERIMENT 1 (24 HOURS)

coccus infection. Similar results shown in Table 58 and Fig. 13 were obtained when the experiment was conducted over a period of five days.

In view of the above observations an investigation was conducted to determine the following: (1) the duration of the apparent increase in resistance which appears to be the result of the prophylactic treatment of animals with the splenic tissue extract SSBK-2; and (2) whether such an induced resistance was associated with a continued or prolonged high serum properdin level in animals that had received treatment with the splenic tissue extract SSBK-2.

In order to establish more definitely if a relation exists between induced resistance by probiotics to *S. aureus* infections and properdin

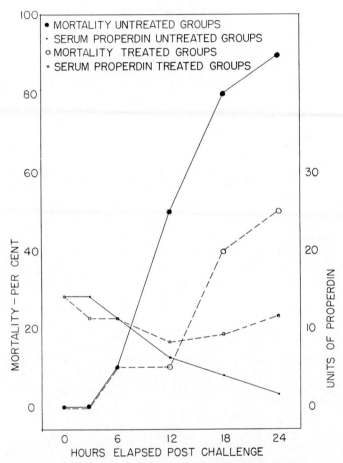

FIG. 12. PERCENT MORTALITY AND SERUM PROPERDIN LEVELS IN
UNTREATED AND SUBCUTANEOUSLY TREATED ANIMALS AFTER
INTRAPERITONEAL CHALLENGE WITH A STANDARDIZED SUSPENSION
OF *Staphylococcus aureus*. EXPERIMENT 2 (24 HOURS)

level, a series of experiments was conducted over an extended period
after treatments with SSKB-2 were initiated.

It was necessary to conduct the following series of preliminary experiments in order to determine the duration of the resistance induced by the
injection of the probiotics.

Adult female Boontucky white mice, 8–9 weeks old and ranging in
weight from 20–25 gm were divided into several groups:

Series A, consisting of 80 mice, received a subcutaneous injection of

TABLE 58

THE PERCENT MORTALITY AND SERUM PROPERDIN LEVELS IN UNTREATED AND
SUBCUTANEOUSLY TREATED ANIMALS AFTER INTRAPERITONEAL CHALLENGE
WITH A STANDARDIZED SUSPENSION OF *Staphylococcus aureus*

Number of Animals	Hours Post-challenge	% Mortality		Units Properdin/Ml	
		Untreated	Treated	Untreated	Treated
10	0	0	0	12	14
10	12	40	30	8	6
20	24	80	40	3	14
20	48	80	40	8	22
20	72	80	40	12	18
20	96	80	40	14	15
20	120	80	40	12	15

100 mg of the splenic tissue extract SSBK-2 in the ventral abdominal
region 24 hr prior to challenge with the organism, S. *aureus* "Grey strain."
Survivors from this series were successively rechallenged at intervals
of 4, 8, and 12 weeks in order to observe the effect of treatment on the
resistance of the animals to successive challenge doses of the organisms.

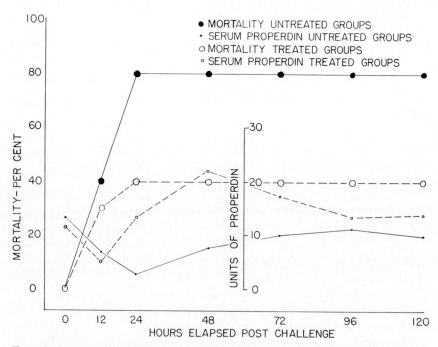

FIG. 13. PERCENT MORTALITY AND SERUM PROPERDIN LEVELS IN UNTREATED AND
SUBCUTANEOUSLY TREATED ANIMALS AFTER INTRAPERITONEAL CHALLENGE WITH A
STANDARDIZED SUSPENSION OF *Staphylococcus aureus*. FIVE DAY EXPERIMENT

Series B, a negative control series consisting of 80 untreated mice, was challenged 24 hr after the injection of 0.5 ml of saline. Survivors from this series were rechallenged after four weeks, with the intent to observe the resistance of the animals to successive challenge doses of the organisms alone, in the absence of prior treatment with the spleen tissue extract SSBK-2.

Series C, a positive control series, consisting of 80 mice treated with the splenic tissue extract as in Series A, was divided into 4 groups of 20 each. These groups were challenged at intervals of 24 hr, 4, 8 and 12 weeks respectively after treatment, so as to coincide with the time of the successive rechallenges of the survivors in Series A and B.

As shown in Table 59, Series A indicates that maximum resistance of

TABLE 59

DURATION OF RESISTANCE TO EXPERIMENTALLY INDUCED *Staphylococcus aureus* INFECTIONS IN MICE BY THE PROPHYLACTIC ADMINISTRATION OF SPLENIC TISSUE EXTRACT SSBK-2

Series	Number of Mice	Interval Between Treatment and Challenge			
		Number of Survivors (%)[1]			
		24 Hours	4 Weeks	8 Weeks	12 Weeks
A. Treatment +	(1)[2] 80	50 (62.5)	35 (70.0)	18 (51.1)	5 (27.7)
successive challenges	(2)[2] 80	52 (65.0)	32 (61.5)	14 (43.7)	2 (14.2)
B. Untreated +	(1) 80	12 (15.0)	0 (0)		
successive challenges	(2) 80	14 (17.5)	0 (0)		
C. Treatment +	(1) 20	12 (60.0)			
single challenge	(2) 20	13 (65.0)			
	(1) 20		12 (60.0)		
	(2) 20		12 (60.0)		
	(1) 20			9 (45.0)	
	(2) 20			7 (35.0)	
	(1) 20				3 (15.0)
	(2) 20				2 (10.0)

[1] Percent survivors calculated on the basis of the number of animals challenged at the various time intervals.

[2] (1) and (2) represent the results of the two separate experiments.

the experimental animals to repeated infection with *S. aureus*, is maintained for a period of four weeks. This resistance is slightly lowered by the eighth week after treatment, but when compared to the negative control Series B, is still relatively high. However by the twelfth week, at the fourth challenge, the resistance has dropped and approximates that of the control animals (Series B) at the time of their primary challenge. The untreated mice in Series B apparently did not acquire any resistance from the primary challenge, since the survivors (15%) succumbed to the second challenge dose of the organisms. This of course prevented further rechallenges. The data of Series C, the positive control, indicate that the resistance effected by prophylactic treatment with the splenic tissue extract SSBK-2 is of a high order (60.0% to 65.0%) gradually decreasing and in close agreement with that observed in Series A (62.5% to 65.0%).

From these results it was apparent that resistance to experimentally induced staphylococcal infections in mice persisted for a period of eight weeks by prophylactic treatment with the splenic tissue extract SSBK-2. This induced resistance, however, was gradually lost 12 weeks after treatment with the extract.

Having established that resistance to induced staphylococcal infections in mice could persist for a period lasting from 8 to 12 weeks by the prophylactic treatment of animals with the splenic tissue extract SSBK-2 the possible relation between resistance established by probiotics and properdin level was limited to the original four-week test period.

Essentially the experiment planned to gain an insight into the existence of such a relationship was patterned along lines similar to those of the preceding work (Table 59), except for the addition of two series of animals "D" and "E." Series D consisted of animals which had received a single treatment dose only, while Series E was challenged once without prior treatment with the tissue extract. In addition to recording the percent survivors within each of the series (A, B, C and E) 24 hr after challenge with a suspension of S. aureus as was done in the previous experiment, this investigation included the determination of the serum properdin levels in each of the Series (A, B, C, D and E) both before and after challenge over the duration of the experiment. The results of these determinations are given in Table 60.

Table 61 shows the mean properdin levels in the experimental animals under various conditions. It has been included to help facilitate the reader in obtaining the overall picture of the results presented in this chapter. It is evident that treatment alone with the splenic tissue extract SSBK-2 appears to have no appreciable effect in either raising or lowering the established mean normal serum properdin level in the experimental animal over a period of 24 hr subsequent to treatment. On the other hand, the results of challenging the experimental animal with a suspension of S. aureus, appeared to bring about a definite lowering of the serum properdin level to approximately $\frac{1}{4}$ the mean normal level, over the 24-hr period following challenge, and subsequently reaching the normal values within 4 to 5 days after challenge. There are indications that this initial drop in properdin titer is associated with a relatively pronounced increase in the mortality rate and in the bacterial viable count of the pooled peritoneal exudates of the untreated animals. Whether in fact such an inter-relationship does exist is subject to specula-

TABLE 60

CORRELATION BETWEEN LASTING RESISTANCE TO STAPHYLOCOCCAL INFECTIONS AND ELEVATED SERUM PROPERDIN LEVELS IN MICE

	(A) Treatment + Successive Challenges	(B) Untreated + Successive Challenges	(C) Treatment + Single Challenge of Separate Groups at Intervals of 4 Weeks Apart	(D) Single Treatment Dose	(E) Single Challenge Dose
Total Number of Mice	175	250	65	20	100
Serum properdin per ml prior to 1st challenge	12	14	10	12	12
No. of mice 1st challenge	170	245	10		95
No. of survivors 24 hr after 1st challenge (%)[1]	106 (62.3)	51 (20.8)	6 (60.0)		18 (18.9)
Serum properdin per ml 24 hr after 1st challenge	10	6	14		4
Serum properdin per ml in survivors prior to 2nd challenge 4 weeks	14	12	12	14	12
No. of mice 2nd challenge	94	40	10		
No. of survivors 24 hr after 2nd challenge (%)[1]	48 (54.2)	9 (22.5)	5 (50.0)		
Serum properdin per ml 24 hr after 2nd challenge	12	5	15		
Serum properdin per ml in survivors prior to 3rd challenge 8 weeks	15	14	14	10	12
No. of mice 3rd challenge	36		10		
No. of survivors 24 hr after 3rd challenge (%)[1]	17 (42.2)		4 (40.0)		
Serum properdin per ml 24 hr after 3rd challenge	10		12		
Serum properdin per ml in survivors prior to 4th challenge 12 weeks	12		12	12	10
No. of mice 4th challenge	7		10		
No. of survivors 24 hr after 4th challenge (%)[1]	2 (28.5)		2 (20.0)		

[1] Percent survivors calculated on the basis of the number of animals challenged at the various time intervals.

TABLE 61

MEAN SERUM PROPERDIN LEVELS PER MILLILITER IN BOONTUCKY
WHITE MICE UNDER VARIOUS CONDITIONS

Groups	Units Properdin per Ml
Normal Boontucky white mice (non-treated, non-challenged)	12.5 (± 1.5)[1](0.06)[2]
Boontucky white mice 24 hr after sub-cutaneous treatment with Spleen Tissue Extract SSBK-2	12.6 (± 1.1)[1](0.05)[2]
Boontucky white mice 24 hr after challenge with a standardized suspension of *Staphylococcus aureus*	3.3 (± 1.3)[1](0.03)[2]

[1] Standard deviation.
[2] Standard error.

tion, especially when it is taken into account that all determinations were conducted on the surviving animals of the individual experiments.

Under conditions of prophylactic treatment followed by challenge, the properdin titer falls to approximately ½ the normal value 12 hr after challenge and then begins a return to normal within the next 12 hr, reaching normal values 24 hr postchallenge. This elevation in the serum properdin level, which differentiates the treated animals from the untreated groups continues, reaching a maximum value 48 hr after inoculation, and then gradually declines, returning to the normal range within 4 to 5 days.

It is apparent that treatment prior to challenge, though not preventing the initial drop in properdin level, restricts the continued and progressive fall in titer which occurs during the first 24 hr after challenge in the absence of treatment, and in addition appears to initiate a possible indirect effect on the host, which manifests itself in a gradual elevation of the serum properdin titers to a maximum of one and one-half times that of the normal range 48 hr after challenge (Table 58 and Fig. 13); it then declines to the normal values within 4 to 5 days.

Summary

The possibility that a nonspecific factor, such as properdin being involved in the resistance to induced staphylococcal infections has been investigated. From the results it appears that the effect of the extract, as related to host resistance, cannot be attributed to a direct stimulation of serum properdin in the experimental animal. It may be related to an indirect effect which, though not clearly identified, manifests itself as a part of the host's defense mechanism in a prevention of the complete depletion of properdin within the first 24 hr of the onset of infection, during which period the animals appear to be most susceptible to the infecting agent. Resistance to repeated challenge of the experimental animal with suspensions of S. *aureus* lasts from between 8 to 12 weeks as a result of a single prophylactic treatment with the splenic tissue extract, and this resistance is independent of a continuous and prolonged elevation of the serum properdin titer over the test period.

DISTRIBUTION AND GROWTH OF BACTERIA IN THE HOST

Previous experiments testing the effect of brain extract and some related pure compounds on the ordinary immune mechanisms as well as on the properdin system did not reveal any significant information on the mechanism of action of probiotics. Therefore, further studies were conducted from a entirely different standpoint.

It has long been known that an essential element in the pathogenicity of any organism is its ability to multiply within tissues of an infected host. Quantitatively or qualitatively virulence can be measured in terms of severity and duration of symptoms and lesions and, ultimately, survival time and mortality. Determination of the bacterial population both in the blood and organs of experimental animals injected with a known lethal dose of staphylococci may also be indicative of the organisms' virulence as well as its behavior.

Nothing is known as to the ability of probiotics to affect the spread of bacteria, their multiplication, their ability to survive as well as their ability to exert toxic effects *in vivo*. The present work is confined to a study of the effect of one of the compounds isolated in small quantities from brain extract, viz., homocarnosine, which, it will be recalled, we have shown to be effective against S. *aureus* prophylactically. The population of staphylococci in the blood stream as well as in organs including kidney, spleen, liver, and lung of experimentally infected control mice is compared with that of mice similarly infected but treated with homocarnosine. The method of Fenner *et al.* (1949), McCune *et al.* (1956), Michael and Massell (1968), Pierce *et al.* (1953), and Smith (1956) was used to quantitate the survival of staphylococci in mouse blood and tissues.

Materials and Methods

The "Original" strain of staphylococci was used in all experiments. It was injected in a volume of 0.5 ml containing 2×10^8 organisms. Mice used in these experiments were females ranging in age from 5 to 9 weeks. They were of the Swiss strain, originally obtained from the Texas Inbred Mice Company. The experimental animals were treated with a total of 5.0 mg of homocarnosine sulphate in 0.25 ml TC Tyrode solution administered in 2 equal doses, one 2 hr before and one 4 hr after subcutaneous challenge with the organism.

Collection of Blood and Determination of Viable Staphylococcal Count.—Blood was collected from all experimental and control animals with heparinized blood hematocrit capillary tubes, by the intraorbital technique. Petri dishes containing SA 110 media were inoculated with a specific amount of blood, and viable counts using the Quebec colony counter, were made after 24 hr incubation. Population of organisms was recorded in terms of number per milliliter of blood.

Preparation of Tissue Homogenates.—All mice were sacrificed with chloroform, and aseptic techniques utilized in removing organs. Tissues were prepared for bacteriological analysis by grinding the organs in a Teflon homogenizer with 5 ml of TC Tyrode solution, and emulsifying with mortar and pestle. In each experiment at least three dilutions of organ emulsions were plated out. The first dilution consisted of the homogenate diluted with 95 ml of sterile distilled water; the second, a tenfold dilution; and the third, a hundredfold dilution. The expression of the organisms in the different organs was based on the number of organisms per weight of organ in grams.

Enumeration of Viable Staphylococci in Organs.—The number of living staphylococci present in the infecting inoculum and the homogenates of tissues of infected animals, both treated and untreated, was determined from plate counts by inoculating SA 110 media with appropriate dilutions of the various suspensions. Colony counts of the organs of treated and untreated infected animals were routinely performed 24 and 72 hr after plate incubation. To minimize personal errors, all counts were made by two independent observers. Utilizing the dilution factors previously described and the number of colonies counted, calculations of the total number of colonies (expressed as viable units of staphylococci per gram of tissue) were determined. These numbers were plotted on logarithm paper as a function of the time after initiation of infection, and the resultant curves taken to represent the fate of the staphylococci in the various organs during the natural course of infection. Each point on the curve represents the mean of the organism population from the tissues of the organs of 3 to 6 animals.

Results

Staphylococcal Population in the Blood of Mice after Infection.— In a series of experiments in which approximately 2×10^8 staphylococci were injected into mice subcutaneously, a reproducible pattern of blood clearance curves was obtained from control animals. An initial fall in bacterial count was seen after 20 to 30 min which was followed by an increase in the count up to 4 hr. Five hours after challenge the count had significantly declined, but small numbers of organisms were still present after 3 days. When 2.5 mg of homocarnosine were injected into mice 2 hr before, followed by 2.5 mg 4 hr after a challenge inoculation of the organism, slight differences between treated and control counts were observed. This was particularly true of the initial decline in bacterial count after 20 min, and the secondary decline after 5 hr in the control group.

In a second group of mice, in which a dosage of 5 mg of homocarnosine was given prophylactically only, at 2 hr prior to challenge of organism, the clearance pattern was similar to that of the control group. However, in neither group of experimental animals does this difference between experimental and control appear to be significant. The results are summarized in Table 62.

As can be seen, in both control and experimental animals, organisms appeared in the blood stream in fairly large numbers 5 min after the organisms were inoculated subcutaneously and were present in relatively the same proportions until the conclusion of the experiment on the third day when they reached a comparative lower level.

It was apparent from these results that homocarnosine definitely did not appear to have its effect through localization of the organism at the site of injection.

TABLE 62

EFFECT OF HOMOCARNOSINE ON THE APPEARANCE AND CLEARANCE OF STAPHYLOCOCCI IN THE BLOOD

| Time After Infection | Number of Viable Organisms per Ml of Blood (x10^2) | | |
| | Control | Experimental | |
		Group 1[1]	Group 2[2]
5 Min	32.0	31.3	51.9
10 Min	82.2	70.4	71.8
20 Min	19.4	105.6	64.2
30 Min	12.3	73.7	35.5
1 Hr	53.4	56.4	50.7
2 Hr	54.5	46.0	82.0
3 Hr	70.0	46.7	65.7
4 Hr	86.2	84.9	70.3
5 Hr	13.6	48.1	17.1
6 Hr	3.6	64.4	4.1
1 Day	1.4	12.8	3.2
2 Days	0.8	1.4	2.4
3 Days	0.5	0.3	0.1

[1] Mice were given a total of 5 mg of homocarnosine 2 hr before and 4 hr after challenge of organism.
[2] Mice were given a total of 5 mg of homocarnosine once only, 2 hr before challenge of organism.

Staphylococcal Population in the Organs of Mice after Infection

Untreated Animals.—Twenty-four hours after the initiation of infection, 50 to 60% of the untreated animals were dead, but the mortality rose only slightly thereafter and ceased at 96 hr. Skin lesions appeared in the survivors as early as 6 days after infection and increased in size until the 14th day after which they gradually decreased. Although the infection did not produce gross lesions, in the present experiments many of the organs, including the spleen and liver, showed an increase in size.

In Fig. 14 may be seen the typical behavior of the staphylococcal population in the kidneys, spleen, liver, and lungs of untreated mice over the 21-day period of observation in these experiments.

It is interesting to note that on the first day after infection, the organism population in the spleens and livers was lower than that in the kidneys, but by the second day both had risen above that of the kidneys. The bacterial count of all organs fluctuated, showing both increases and decreases in the first week of infection, after which there was a period

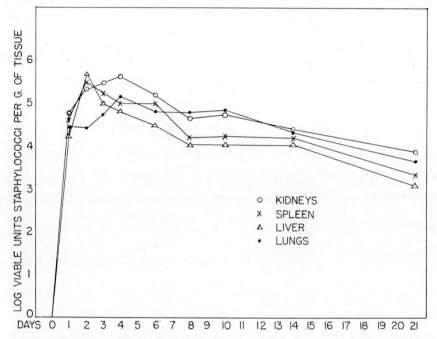

FIG. 14. POPULATION OF *Staphylococcus aureus* IN ORGANS OF UNTREATED ANIMALS
AS FUNCTION OF TIME

of gradual stabilization of the population census in all organs and eventually a slow decline. In general, these latter two phases closely paralleled one another for all four organs, but the counts for the spleen and liver were slightly lower than those for the kidneys and lungs. At the end of 21 days, however, the count in all organs continued to be substantial.

Treated Animals.—In Table 63 are the comparative values of the counts of the organisms in the organs of treated and untreated animals taken at various time intervals during the course of the experiments. Since all of the accompanying graphs (Fig. 15, 16, 17 and 18) are plotted on log paper it was felt that a knowledge of the actual number of organisms might be of aid to the reader in evaluating the results. It is to be noted that from both the Table and the 4 illustrations there are 1- and 2-day postinfection organism counts and log units for all organs of

TABLE 63

COMPARISON OF THE STAPHYLOCOCCAL POPULATION IN THE KIDNEYS, SPLEEN, LIVER AND LUNGS OF UNTREATED ANIMALS AND ANIMALS TREATED WITH 5 MG OF HOMOCARNOSINE

Untreated Animals: Organs Removed from Survivors

Day	Kidneys	Spleen	Liver	Lungs
1	88,000[1]	67,000	29,000	31,000
2	420,000	470,000	580,000	31,000
3	429,000	273,000	127,000	85,000
4	465,000	131,000	49,000	138,000
6	160,000	120,000	47,000	89,000
8	63,000	25,000	16,000	70,000
10	72,000	31,000	22,000	73,000
14	31,000	16,000	13,000	24,000
21	15,000	8,000	7,000	12,000

Untreated Animals: Organs Removed from Dead Animals Shortly After Death

Day	Kidneys	Spleen	Liver	Lungs
1	3,800,000	1,640,000	840,000	230,000
2	4,000,000	7,900,000	2,900,000	150,000

Treated Animals: Organs Removed from Survivors

Day	Kidneys	Spleen	Liver	Lungs
1	23,600	8,900	3,600	4,300
2	47,000	55,000	12,000	21,000
3	59,000	10,000	9,000	30,000
4	29,000	14,000	17,000	10,000
6	22,000	18,000	17,000	39,000
8	13,000	18,000	11,000	11,000
10	14,000	17,000	10,000	32,000
14	4,100	3,300	400	3,500
21	100	0	0	100

[1] Numbers indicate population of organisms per gram of tissue.

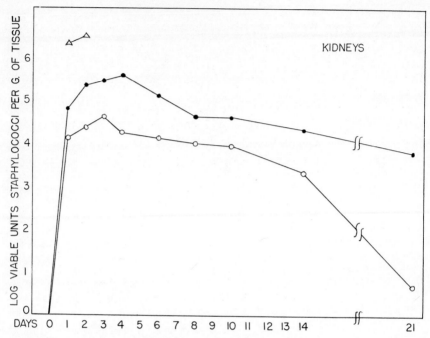

FIG. 15. COMPARISON OF *Staphylococcus aureus* POPULATION IN KIDNEYS OF TREATED
AND UNTREATED ANIMALS AS FUNCTION OF TIME

△ ———— △ Counts in Control Animals Dying from Infection;
● ———— ● Counts in Control Animals Surviving Infection;
○ ———— ○ Counts in Experimental Animals Treated with Homocarnosine.

untreated animals which died of their infection. All other illustrations,
both for treated and untreated animals, were derived from animals
which were living and were sacrificed for this purpose.

As can be seen from both the illustrations and the Table, neither
the treated nor untreated surviving animals attain counts approaching
those of the untreated dead animals. Apparently the number of organisms
entering the organs from the blood stream is very important in determining the ultimate mortality of the animals, even though the number
entering the different organs varies considerably. It may be noted that
the number of organisms in the lungs is particularly low as compared
with that of the other organs. Furthermore, it can be seen that throughout the course of infection the bacterial count in the various organs of
the treated animals is always below that of the untreated. It would
appear possible that it is this difference in the number of organisms
entering the organs that accounts for the margin of safety provided by

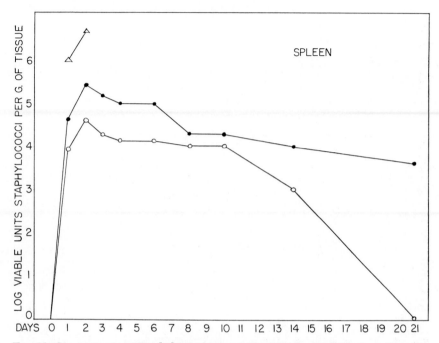

FIG. 16. COMPARISON OF *Staphylococcus aureus* POPULATION IN SPLEEN OF TREATED
AND UNTREATED ANIMALS AS FUNCTION OF TIME

△————△ Counts in Control Animals Dying from Infection;
●————● Counts in Control Animals Surviving Infection;
○————○ Counts in Experimental Animals Treated with Homocarnosine.

homocarnosine in these experiments, and particularly in those in which
the number of infecting organisms is high.

Another finding well-illustrated in the figures is the striking difference
which occurs in the organ population of the treated animals at about
the tenth day following infection. At this time there is a marked decline
in the bacteria count in the organs of the treated animals as compared
to the untreated, particularly that of the spleen and liver. After 14 days,
the decline was greatly accelerated in all the organs of the treated
animals and by the 21st day the spleen and liver were completely free of
organisms, and only a few remained in the kidney and lungs.

As previously stated, it would appear that homocarnosine may act by
effecting a decrease in the number of bacteria entering the organs. It is
highly improbable that this decrease is due to any such effect as phagocy-
tosis which might occur in the blood stream since the white blood cells
are, for all practical purposes, only slightly phagocytic while in the cir-

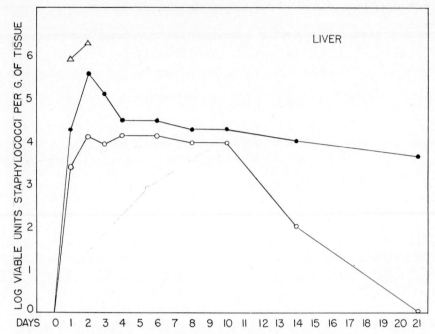

FIG. 17. COMPARISON OF *Staphylococcus aureus* POPULATION IN LIVER OF TREATED
AND UNTREATED ANIMALS AS FUNCTION OF TIME

△——————△ Counts in Control Animals Dying from Infection;
●——————● Counts in Control Animals Surviving Infection;
○——————○ Counts in Experimental Animals Treated with Homocarnosine.

culatory system. The mechanism responsible for the failure of the
organisms in treated animals to enter the organ in sufficient numbers
to produce death is apparently due to some tissue factor which as yet
we have been unable to explain.

REFERENCES

BRANDIS, H. 1954. Part 3. On proimmunity (depression immunity). Ergebn.
    Hyg. Bact. Immunitatforsch. und Exp. Therap. 28, 141.
FENNER, F., MARTIN, S. P., and PIERCE, C. H. 1949. The enumeration of
    viable tubercle bacilli in cultures and infected tissues. Ann. N.Y. Acad. Sci.
    52, 751–764.
KAHN, R. L. 1934. Tissue reactions in immunity. XIV. The specific reacting
    capacities of different tissues of an immunized animal. Science 79, 172–175.
KAHN, R. L. 1936. Tissue Immunity. Chas. C Thomas, Springfield, Ill.
KAHN, R. L., BLATT, I. M., and KIM, S. H. 1956. Studies on tissue reactions
    in immunity, XVIII. Local response of mid-facial and other areas of im-

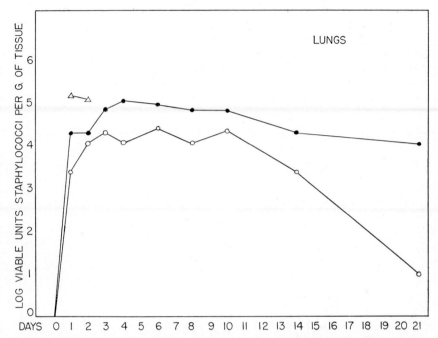

FIG. 18. COMPARISON OF *Staphylococcus aureus* POPULATION IN LUNGS OF TREATED
AND UNTREATED ANIMALS AS FUNCTION OF TIME

△————△ Counts in Control Animals Dying from Infection;
●————● Counts in Control Animals Surviving Infection;
○————○ Counts in Experimental Animals Treated with Homocarnosine.

munized rabbits to subcutaneous injections of protein antigen. Univ. Mich.
Med. Bull. 22, 73–79.

KOLLE, W., and PRIGGE, R. 1929. Cholera asiatica. *In* Handbook of Pathogenic
Microorganisms, W. Kolle, R. Kraus, and P. Uhlenhuth (Editors) 1, 623.

LANDSTEINER, K. 1945. The Specificity of Serological Reactions, 2nd Edition.
Harvard Univ. Press, Cambridge, Mass.

McCUNE, R. M., JR., DINEEN, P. O. P., and BATTEN, J. C. 1956. The effect
of antimicrobial drugs on an experimental staphylococcal infection in mice.
In Staphylococcal infections. I. Host factors in experimental staphylococcal
infections. Ann. N.Y. Acad. Sci. 65, 91–102.

MICHAEL, J. G., and MASSELL, B. F. 1968. Dynamics in development of experimental streptococcal immunity in mice. J. Bacteriol. 96, 131–138.

OSBORNE, T. W. B. 1937. Complement or Ataxin. Oxford Univ. Press, London.

PIERCE, C. H., DUBOS, R. J., and SCHAEFER, W. B. 1953. Multiplication and
survival of tubercle bacilli in the organs of mice. J. Exptl. Med. 97, 189–206.

PILLEMER, L. 1943. Recent advances in the chemistry of complement. Chem.
Rev. 33, 1–26.

PILLEMER, L. 1955. The properdin system. Trans. N.Y. Acad. Sci. 17, 526.

PILLEMER, L. *et al.* 1954A. The properdin system and immunity. I. Demonstration and isolation of a new serum protein, properdin, and the role in immune phenomena. Science *120*, 279–285.

PILLEMER, L. *et al.* 1954B. The properdin system and immunity. I. Demonstration and isolation of a new serum protein, properdin, and the role in immune phenomena. Federation Proc. *13*, 508.

PILLEMER, L., SCHOENBERG, M. D., BLUM, L., and WURZ, L. 1955. Properdin system and immunity. II. Interaction of the properdin system with polysaccharides. Science *122*, 545–549.

ROWLEY, D. 1955. Stimulation of natural immunity to *Escherichia coli* infections. Observations on mice. Lancet *I*, 232–234 Jan. 29, 1955.

SMITH, J. M. 1956. Studies on the fate of virulent and avirulent staphylococci in mice. Ann. N.Y. Acad. Sci. *65*, 67–72.

ZINSSER, J., ENDERS, J. P., and FOTHERGILL, L. D. 1946. Immunity Principles and Application in Medicine and Public Health. Macmillan Co., New York.

Index